Emergency
Ultrasound

MADE EASY

Edited by

Justin Bowra MBBS FACEM CCPU

Director of Emergency Medicine Training, Sydney Adventist Hospital;
Senior Emergency Physician, Royal North Shore and Sydney Adventist Hospitals;
Senior Lecturer, University of Notre Dame Australia, Sydney, Australia

Russell E McLaughlin MB BCH BAO FRCSI MMedSci FCEM CFEU

Clinical Director, Emergency Department, Royal Victoria Hospital, Belfast, UK

Second edition

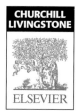

Edinburgh London New York Oxford Philadelphia St Louis Sydney Toronto 2011

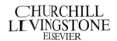

CHURCHILL
LIVINGSTONE
ELSEVIER

First edition 2006
Second edition 2011
Reprinted 2013 (three times), 2014

ISBN 9780702041907

British Library Cataloguing in Publication Data
A catalogue record for this book is available from the British Library

Library of Congress Cataloging in Publication Data
A catalog record for this book is available from the Library of Congress

Notices
Knowledge and best practice in this field are constantly changing. As new research and experience broaden our understanding, changes in research methods, professional practices, or medical treatment may become necessary.

Practitioners and researchers must always rely on their own experience and knowledge in evaluating and using any information, methods, compounds, or experiments described herein. In using such information or methods they should be mindful of their own safety and the safety of others, including parties for whom they have a professional responsibility.

With respect to any drug or pharmaceutical products identified, readers are advised to check the most current information provided (i) on procedures featured or (ii) by the manufacturer of each product to be administered, to verify the recommended dose or formula, the method and duration of administration, and contraindications. It is the responsibility of practitioners, relying on their own experience and knowledge of their patients, to make diagnoses, to determine dosages and the best treatment for each individual patient, and to take all appropriate safety precautions.

To the fullest extent of the law, neither the publisher nor the authors, contributors, or editors, assume any liability for any injury and/or damage to persons or property as a matter of products liability, negligence or otherwise, or from any use or operation of any methods, products, instructions, or ideas contained in the material herein.

ELSEVIER your source for books,
journals and multimedia
in the health sciences

www.elsevierhealth.com

Working together to grow
libraries in developing countries

www.elsevier.com | www.bookaid.org | www.sabre.org

ELSEVIER   BOOK AID International   Sabre Foundation

The publisher's policy is to use paper manufactured from sustainable forests

Printed in China

Emergency
Ultrasound
MADE EASY

Commissioning Editor: Laurence Hunter
Development Editor: Helen Leng
Project Manager: Glenys Norquay/Kerrie-Anne McKinlay
Designer/Design Direction: Charles Gray
Illustration Manager: Bruce Hogarth
Illustrator: Graham Chambers

Contents

Contents

Contributors

Paul Atkinson MB MA(CANTAB) MRCP FCEM CFEU
Associate Professor, Dalhousie University;
Director of Research, Department of
Emergency Medicine, Saint John Regional
Hospital, Saint John, Canada

Roslyn E Bell BSC MB BCH BAO FRCR
Consultant Radiologist, Antrim Area
Hospital, Antrim, UK

Michael Blaivas MD
Professor, Emergency and Internal
Medicine, Northside Hospital Forsyth,
Atlanta, USA

Justin Bowra MBBS FACEM CCPU
Director of Emergency Medicine Training,
Sydney Adventist Hospital; Senior
Emergency Physician, Royal North, Shore
and Sydney Adventist Hospitals; Senior
Lecturer, University of Notre Dame,
Sydney, Australia

Niall Collum MRCS(ED) FCEM
Consultant, Emergency Medicine, Ulster
Hospital, Belfast, UK

Anthony P Joseph FACEM
Clinical Associate Professor, Sydney
Medical School, University of Sydney,
Senior Staff Specialist, Emergency;
Department and Director of Trauma, Royal
North Shore Hospital, Sydney, Australia

Andrew W Kirkpatrick CD MD MHSC FRCSC FACS
Medical Director Regional Trauma
Services, Foothills Medical Centre, Calgary,
Canada

Sabrina Kuah FRANZCOG
Consultant Obstetrician, Department of
Perinatal Medicine, Women's and
Children's Hospital, Adelaide, Australia

Stella McGinn PHD FRACP MRCPE
Staff Specialist in Nephrology, Royal North
Shore Hospital; Clinical Senior Lecturer,
Department of Medicine, University of
Sydney, Australia

Russell E McLaughlin MB BCH BAO FRCSI MMEDSCI FCEM CFEU
Clinical Director, Emergency Department,
Royal Victoria Hospital, Belfast, UK

John T McManus MD MCR FACEP FAAEM
LTC(P) Director, US Army Emergency
Medical Service, EMS Fellowship Program
Director, San Antonio Uniformed Services
Health, Education Consortium; Medical
Director Fort Sam Houston and Camp
Bullis Fire Dept; Clinical Associate
Professor, Emergency Medicine, University
of Texas, Heath Science Center, San
Antonio, USA

Robert F Reardon MD
Ultrasound Director, Department of
Emergency Medicine, Hennepin County
Medical Center; Associate Professor,
University of Minnesota, Minneapolis,
USA

Conn Russell FCA DIBICM
Consultant, Anaesthesia and Intensive
Care Medicine, Ulster Hospital, Belfast,
UK

Preface

Ultrasound (US) is a safe, rapid imaging technique. Emergency US is used to answer very specific questions, such as the presence or absence of AAA (abdominal aortic aneurysm), or of free fluid (such as blood) in the abdomen after trauma. Unlike other imaging modalities (e.g. CT scan) it is a rapid technique that can 'come to the patient'. Emergency US is not a substitute for formal US by an appropriately trained radiologist. It has no role in routine situations such as antenatal screening.

Emergency Ultrasound Made Easy is aimed particularly at specialists and trainees in emergency medicine, surgery and intensive care. However, its scope is broad. For example, rapid diagnosis of DVT (deep vein thrombosis) may be of interest to any hospital doctor and AAA screening may be of value in primary care as well as a hospital setting.

There are already many excellent comprehensive textbooks of ultrasound, and this book is not designed as such. As a pocket-sized handbook of emergency US, this book provides a rapid guide to its use and interpretation. It is designed to be accessible and easy to use in an urgent situation (e.g. a shocked trauma patient).

In the five years since the first edition of *Emergency Ultrasound Made Easy* there have been major advances in the practice of emergency medicine and related disciplines, and this edition has been comprehensively revised and updated to reflect these advances. They have occurred owing to the pioneering efforts of individual clinicians and also the rapidly evolving technology that has made high-quality portable imaging widely available.

Despite the fact that the debate of radiology versus non-radiology is over and ultrasound is a 'tool for everyone', this edition still firmly adheres to the principles of only using ultrasound where it adds value and only asking simple questions that may be readily addressed using ultrasound. The core paradigm of 'Yes', 'No' or 'Don't know' still applies and the practitioner asking these questions must be engaged in a robust quality-assurance process.

Justin Bowra & Russell McLaughlin

Acknowledgements

To our wives Stella McGinn and Ros Bell whose patience and good humour made this possible! To our children Niamh Bowra, Matthew McLaughlin and Jacob McLaughlin. We have no plans to write 'Raising Children Made Easy'.

Thanks to Dr Sanjeeva Abeywickrema, Consultant Radiologist, St George's Hospital, Sydney.

Abbreviations

AAA	abdominal aortic aneurysm	**LA**	local anaesthetic
AP	anteroposterior	**LMP**	last menstrual period
ARF	acute renal failure	**LP**	lumbar puncture
ASIS	anterior superior iliac spine	**LS**	longitudinal section
ATLS®	Advanced Trauma Life Support	**LV**	left ventricle (or left ventricular)
βHCG	beta human chorionic gonadotrophin	**MRI**	magnetic resonance imaging
		MSD	mean sac diameter
BP	blood pressure	**NICE**	National Institute for Health and Clinical Excellence
CBD	common bile duct		
CCA	common carotid artery	**OG**	obstetrics and gynaecology (or obstetricians and gynaecologists)
CCF	congestive cardiac failure		
CT	computed tomography		
CTKUB	computed tomography of kidneys, ureter and bladder	**OR**	odds ratio
		OT	operating theatre
CVC	central vein cannula *or* central venous cannulation	**PE**	pulmonary embolism *or* embolus
		PEA	pulseless electrical activity
CVP	central venous pressure	**PLAX**	parasternal long axis
CXR	chest X-ray	**PTX**	pneumothorax
DPL	diagnostic peritoneal lavage	**PV**	portal vein
DVT	deep vein thrombosis	**PZT**	piezo-electric transducer
ED	emergency department	**RV**	right ventricle (or right ventricular)
EFAST	extended focused assessment with sonography in trauma		
		SA	subclavian artery
EP	ectopic pregnancy	**SCFE**	slipped capital femoral epiphysis
FAST	focused assessment with sonography in trauma		
		SCM	sternocleidomastoid muscle
FB	foreign body	**SMA**	superior mesenteric artery
FF	free fluid	**SPC**	suprapubic catheter
FHB	foetal heart beat	**TA**	transabdominal
FHR	foetal heart rate	**TS**	transverse section
FN	femoral nerve	**TV**	transvaginal
FV	femoral vein	**TVS**	transvaginal ultrasound
GA	gestational age	**UA**	ulnar artery
GB	gallbladder	**UN**	ulnar nerve
ICC	intercostal catheter	**US**	ultrasound
IJV	internal jugular vein	**VB**	vertebral body
IUP	*in utero* pregnancy	**WES**	wall-echo shadow
IVC	inferior vena cava		

1 Introduction

Justin Bowra, Russell McLaughlin

What is ultrasound?

Diagnostic ultrasound (US) is a safe, rapid imaging technique. It is non-invasive and painless, requires no contrast media and no special patient preparation for routine studies. US is used widely by radiologists, cardiologists (echocardiography) and obstetricians. In recent years its use has become widespread in the field of critical care (emergency medicine, intensive care and anaesthetics). This edition of *Emergency Ultrasound Made Easy* has been comprehensively updated to reflect the latest advances in critical care US.

What is emergency US?

Emergency US, also known as emergency bedside ultrasound (EBU), limited US or focused US, is a modification of US performed by non-radiologists. Unlike other imaging modalities (e.g. computed tomography (CT) scan), it is a rapid technique that can 'come to the patient' and be repeated as often as necessary.

It allows rapid bedside identification of certain life-threatening conditions such as:
- abdominal aortic aneurysm (AAA)
- pericardial effusion
- traumatic haemoperitoneum (FAST scan, focused assessment with sonography in trauma)
- pneumothorax (extended FAST, or EFAST).

It also improves the safety of certain procedures by allowing them to be performed under US guidance, such as:
- central vein cannulation
- pericardiocentesis, thoracocentesis, paracentesis
- peripheral nerve blocks
- lumbar puncture
- suprapubic catheter insertion
- soft tissue foreign body removal.

What it isn't (you are not a radiologist!)

Unlike formal US, this technique does not require years of training. Studies have shown that it can be quickly taught and that as few as 10 scans may suffice for an operator to obtain acceptable scans for a given indication.

However, it must be emphasized that it is *not* a substitute for formal US by an appropriately trained radiologist. It has no role in routine situations such as antenatal screening or the diagnosis of breast lumps, for example.

Why is this? Radiologists are trained to scan and interpret images in detail, using an in-depth understanding of the relevant anatomy, pathology and US images of the scanned area. By contrast, emergency US is limited to answering *specific* questions only, and training and credentialing guidelines reflect this.

Furthermore, by its very nature, US is very operator-dependent. Image acquisition and interpretation can be very challenging for the novice, particularly in an emergency. Keep this in mind as you learn how to scan.

First considerations

It is wise to bear in mind the following important principles when training in emergency US.

The clinical question to be answered

Ideally this should have a *binary answer (yes/no)*. For example, 'Does the patient have an aortic aneurysm?' rather than 'What is causing this patient's abdominal pain?' Unlike formal US, emergency US uses a few, clearly defined views to answer binary questions very quickly. An understanding of this concept is absolutely fundamental to safe interpretation of images (Table 1.1).

Asking the wrong question is worse than useless. It is *dangerous* and fails to recognize the limitations of emergency US. For example, a negative FAST scan will lead to false reassurance if you fail to understand that it does not rule out solid organ injury.

Limitations of emergency US

Not all binary questions can be answered. US must be *capable* of answering the clinical question. For example, US is sensitive in the detection of hydronephrosis but is poor at identifying ureteric stones. Therefore, in a patient with suspected

Table 1.1 Binary thinking		
Clinical situation	**The right question (answer: Yes or No)**	**The wrong question(s)**
Severe epigastric pain	Does this patient have AAA?	What is causing the pain? If AAA, is it leaking?
Blunt abdominal trauma (FAST)	Is there free intraperitoneal fluid?	Is there solid organ injury? Is there a viscus rupture?
Painful leg	Is there an above-knee DVT?	What is causing the pain?

AAA = abdominal aortic aneurysm; DVT = deep vein thrombosis; FAST = focused assessment with sonography in trauma.

ureteric colic, the right questions (those US can answer) are:
- Does this patient have AAA (as a differential diagnosis)?
- Does this patient have hydronephrosis (implying obstruction by a calculus)?
- Can I identify a calculus?

The wrong question:
- Can I *exclude* a calculus?

Operator and technical limitations

Some questions are beyond the reach of emergency US. An ultrasonographer using highly specialized equipment can identify pathology not visible to the emergency sonologist using a portable machine. That said, as portable machines continue to improve, this statement may require revision in the future.

Furthermore, when you begin scanning you are not yet an emergency sonologist. The temptation to make clinical decisions based on scan results may be overwhelming for the beginner. However, all new diagnostic and therapeutic techniques require a program of credentialing and ongoing maintenance of standards. Until the operator has achieved a minimum level of experience, great caution must be exercised in the performance and interpretation of emergency US scans for any new indication.

Will a scan change management in the emergency department (ED)?

There is no point performing examinations that are better performed by others unless there is a clear benefit to the patient or the department. For example, it is possible to identify many paediatric limb fractures on US. However, if you are also planning a diagnostic X-ray, then US may cause the patient unnecessary distress.

Similarly, US identification of hydronephrosis matters little if the clinician requires CT to diagnose ureteric colic. However, the finding of hydronephrosis matters a great deal in a patient with acute renal failure as prompt decompression may prevent progression to dialysis.

Summary

➡ Emergency US is rapid, safe, sensitive and allows ongoing resuscitation of the patient in the ED.
➡ It allows rapid (Yes/No) answers to specific binary questions.
➡ It is extremely dependent on operator and equipment limitations.
➡ Like all ED investigations, it is only indicated if it will change management.
➡ It is *not a substitute* for formal US.

2 How ultrasound works

Roslyn E Bell, Russell McLaughlin

What is ultrasound?

Ultrasound (US) uses high-frequency sound waves which are transmitted through the body from a transducer (probe). US waves are of much higher frequency than waves at the limit of human hearing; they usually range from 2 to 15 MHz (1 Hz = 1 cycle/second), with higher frequencies (e.g. 7–12 MHz) used for more superficial scanning, and 3.5–5 MHz transducers most commonly used for abdominal scanning. As frequency increases, resolution improves, but the ability to penetrate to deeper structures decreases (Fig. 2.1).

Types of US

There are several different modes of US, including M-mode used in echocardiography and pleural imaging, B-mode used in abdominal and musculoskeletal scanning, and Doppler imaging used when imaging flowing blood (in conjunction with B-mode).

B-mode scanning is the main mode covered in this text. In this mode the US beam is swept through the patient's body, producing a two-dimensional (2D) scan plane. The tissues are represented on the screen in the form of a myriad of tiny white dots, which together form a 2D image.

In M-mode, a single line of B-mode echoes is continuously updated across the screen. The on-screen horizontal axis represents time, and the vertical axis represents depth. This mode shows movement such as the movement of the pleura when evaluating for pneumothorax.

Producing the image

The US pulses are produced within the transducer (probe) by passing an electromagnetic wave through a piezo-electric crystal causing it to vibrate. After each pulse has been produced the transducer switches to receiving mode. The transducer acts in the receiving mode for most of the time. The waves reflected back from the tissue boundaries cause the crystal to vibrate and produce an electrical signal. The probe's 'matching layer' improves energy transmission (Fig. 2.2).

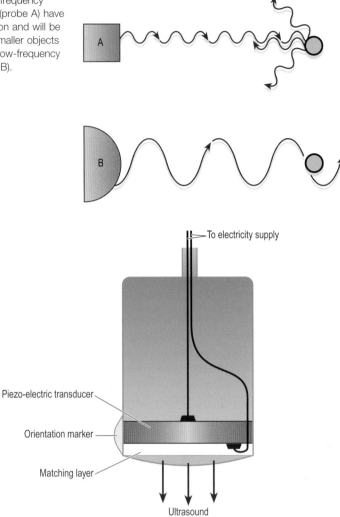

Fig. 2.1 High-frequency sound waves (probe A) have better resolution and will be reflected by smaller objects compared to low-frequency waves (probe B).

To electricity supply

Piezo-electric transducer

Orientation marker

Matching layer

Ultrasound

Fig. 2.2 Probe and orientation marker. The 'matching layer', which is made of epoxy resin, improves energy transmission.

US waves travel at slightly different speeds through different tissues, and are reflected, absorbed or scattered at the boundaries between different media. When US waves hit these boundaries 'echoes' are sent back to the probe and are detected and analysed to form the image. The image on the screen is displayed as a series of dots, and the position of each of these dots depends on the time taken for the echo to return to the transducer. Echoes from deeper tissues take longer to return to the probe and are therefore positioned accordingly on the display. The brightness of each dot corresponds to the echo amplitude. Each US pulse from the transducer produces a series of dots, and many pulses are used to produce a cross-sectional image.

Sound energy travels through different media at different speeds. Approximate values are given in Table 2.1.

Table 2.1 Ultrasound: speed through various media	
Medium	**Speed of sound (metres/second)**
Soft tissue	1570
Bone	3000
Water	1480
Fat	1450
Air	330

Each medium has different impedance to the passage of the sound wave, called its acoustic impedance. The greater the difference in acoustic impedance at a boundary, the greater the reflection of the sound wave.

It is therefore the varying properties and 'textures' of tissues that produce the different echoes, and consequently the differing 'echogenicities' of tissues seen on the image. Some examples (Figs 2.3 and 2.4):

- Bone cortex and calcified gallstones are highly reflective and appear white.
- Fluid (e.g. in bladder) transmits sound waves and appears black.
- Soft tissue (e.g. liver) is part-way between the two and appears grey.

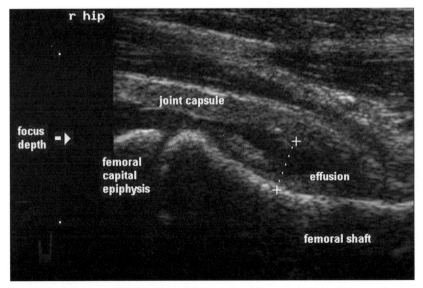

Fig. 2.3 Hip effusion with bone, fluid, soft tissue. Note that the effusion (fluid) appears black. A focus arrow is labelled at the side of the image.

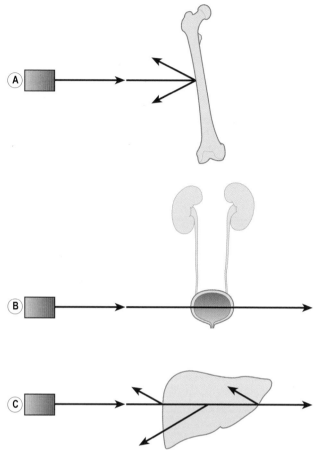

Fig. 2.4 Bone (A) is highly reflective and appears white. Fluid in the bladder (B) transmits sound and appears black. The liver (C), which reflects some sound and transmits the rest, appears grey.

US gel is used between the probe and the patient as a 'coupling' agent because US waves require a transport medium and do not pass well through air.

The transducer

The most commonly used transducers (Fig. 2.5) in modern medical US are linear array and phased array, both of which have a row of small separate piezo-electric transducer (PZT) elements.

Linear array transducers produce a rectangular image, are generally of higher frequency—for example, 7–12 MHz—and are used to produce high-resolution images when scanning superficial and musculoskeletal structures. The PZT elements are activated electronically in sequence.

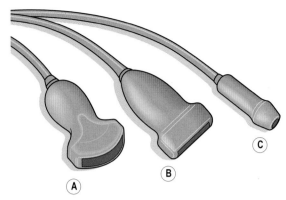

Fig. 2.5 Transducers. (A) Low-frequency curved probe. (B) High-frequency linear array probe. (C) Phased-array microconvex probe.

Curvilinear transducers are essentially linear transducers constructed with a curve. They provide a wider field of view and are more suitable for deeper structures as the most superficial layers are distorted by the curved probe.

Phased array, or sector transducers produce US beams by the PZT elements that are electronically steered by applying the voltage to the elements with small time differences. The beam is therefore swept through the tissues to produce a wide field of view image. These can be used in abdominal scanning and echocardiography, and are useful for areas that require a small 'footprint', for example, between ribs, as the transducer head is usually smaller than that of a curvilinear probe.

Orientation

It is important always to hold the probe in the correct orientation, as this will allow rapid identification of anatomy and the production of reliable and comparable images. On the image the patient's skin is at the top of the screen, and deeper structures towards the bottom of the screen.

When scanning longitudinally (sagittally), the patient's *head* should lie to the left of the screen and feet to the right. A longitudinal scan is shown in Figure 2.6.

When imaging in the transverse plane, the patient's *right side* should lie to the left of the screen. A transverse scan is shown in Figure 2.7.

The probe is usually marked with a small light or other marker at one side, which should point to the patient's head for a longitudinal scan or the patient's right side for a transverse scan (Fig. 2.2). Alternatively, by tapping a finger gently on one side of the probe, the user can check image alignment. Please note that the conventional orientation will be reversed with

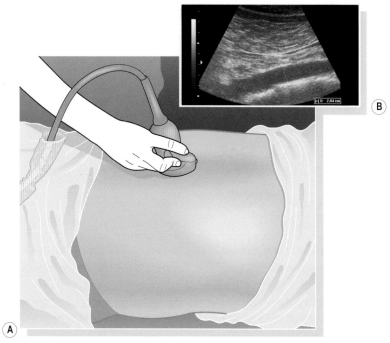

Fig. 2.6 Longitudinal scan. (A) Probe orientation on body. (B) US image showing the upper aorta (in the lower part of the image); note that the blood-filled (i.e. fluid-filled) aorta is darker than the surrounding tissue.

cardiac imaging and this can lead to confusion. What is more important than convention is that the user has a clear understanding of what is observed.

The keyboard

The following are the important knobs (Fig. 2.8) used during a routine emergency department (ED) scan. There may be some variation in the labelling of these knobs on some makes of machine but these are the most commonly used.

Gain

Turning up the gain amplifies the signal from the returning echoes, making the image more white and less dark. At the appropriate gain setting the image should be neither too bright nor too dark, simple fluid should appear black (anechoic), and the distribution should be uniform from top to bottom of the image.

Time gain compensation

This is the set of slide bars on the keyboard that allow adjustment of gain at different levels of the image;

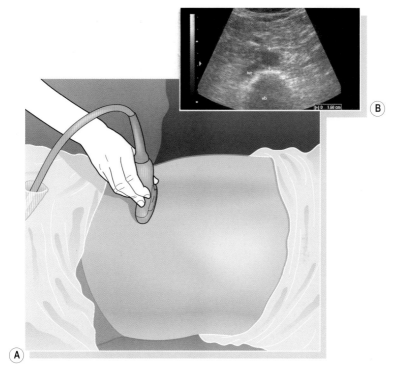

Fig. 2.7 Transverse scan. (A) Probe orientation on body. (B) A cross-section of the lower aorta is shown in the centre of this US image. ivc = inferior vena cava; vb = vertebral body.

for example, deeper layers may need increased gain.

Depth

This increases/decreases the depth of tissue visible; for example, depth is decreased to maximize the image of superficial structures and is increased to visualize deeper structures.

Focus/position

Arrow(s) at the side of the image (Fig. 2.3) designate the focal zone(s). They can be moved to sharpen the image at the level of interest. Many modern machines now have an autofocus that obviates the need to focus manually.

Freeze

This button should be pressed to freeze the image prior to printing or saving the image, or performing measurements.

Artefacts

An artefact is an image, or part of an image, that does not correspond to anatomy at that position in the patient. Artefacts can be useful in the interpretation of an image, or can obscure information. Examples of artefacts include the following.

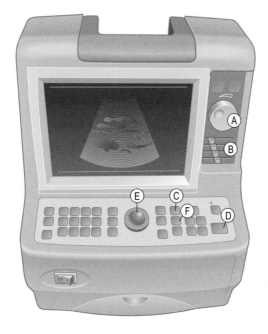

A	Gain
B	Time gain compensation
C	Focus
D	Freeze
E	Master control
F	Depth control

Fig. 2.8 Keyboard, with parts labelled.

Acoustic enhancement and acoustic windows (Fig. 2.9)

Acoustic enhancement occurs when sound energy passes through a fluid-filled structure (e.g. urinary bladder, cysts, blood vessels). More sound energy passes through the tissues and returns to the probe (less attenuation), so tissues behind the fluid appear bright. Hence, the fluid acts as an 'acoustic window' for deeper structures. For example, in pelvic scans, a full bladder acts as an acoustic window to help visualize deeper tissues.

Acoustic shadowing

This is the opposite of acoustic enhancement and occurs when sound energy hits a highly reflective structure (e.g. bone cortex or calculi), leaving little US energy to reach deeper structures. The tissues behind appear dark. This can be useful when scanning the gall bladder as gall-stones can be recognized by their posterior shadow (Fig. 2.10). However, shadowing can be problematic. For example, shadowing caused by ribs in the upper abdomen and chest can obscure deeper structures (Fig. 2.11), and in older people leg veins can be obscured by calcified arteries.

Edge shadows

These are shadows cast by the curved walls of some rounded structures, such as gall bladder or blood vessel,

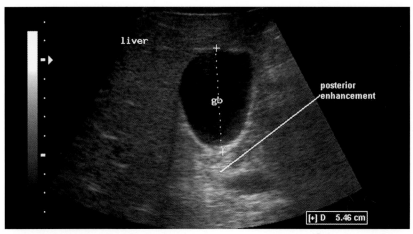

Fig. 2.9 Gall bladder (gb) and posterior acoustic enhancement. (See section 'Acoustic enhancement and acoustic windows'.)

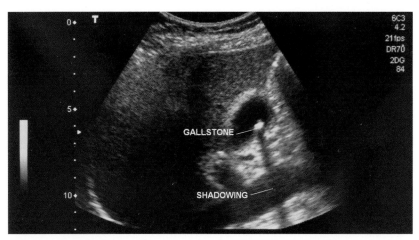

Fig. 2.10 Gallstone with posterior acoustic shadowing. (See section 'Acoustic shadowing'.)

due to strong reflection from the convex surface.

Mirror image (Fig. 2.12)

This is caused by reflection between a structure and a large curved interface. The time of the echo return is delayed, and therefore the on-screen images are placed deeper than their actual location. A 'mirror image' of the structure appears on the other side of the interface; for example, mirror image of bladder in pelvis.

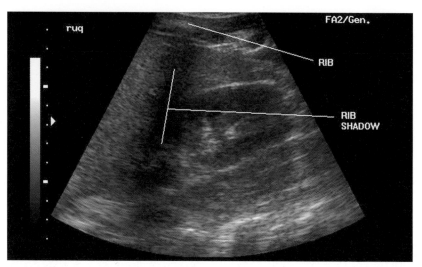

Fig. 2.11 Rib with posterior acoustic shadowing. The rib has shielded deeper structures from sound energy. The ability of acoustic shadowing to obscure deeper structures can be problematic. (See section 'Acoustic shadowing'.)

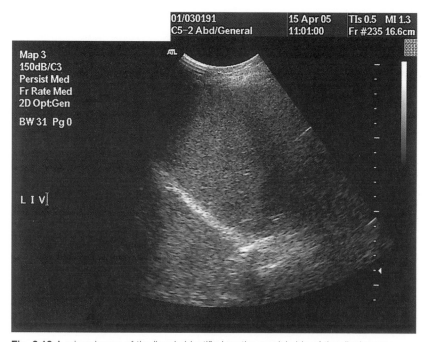

Fig. 2.12 A mirror image of the liver is identified on the cranial side of the diaphragm.

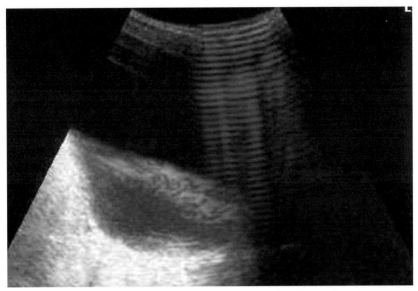

Fig. 2.13 Transverse scan of bladder demonstrating reverberation artefact on right of image.

Reverberation (Fig. 2.13)

This appears as parallel, evenly spaced lines and is caused by multiple sound wave reflections between a structure and the probe or between two structures. The sound wave 'bounces' and returns to the probe more than once, producing an image with each reflection. This can occur if too little gel is used.

Handy hints

✓ When starting work with a new US machine familiarize yourself with the keyboard layout and functions as there is considerable variation between products.

✓ Orientate the probe prior to each scan to avoid confusion:
  ✓ longitudinal scan: patient's *head* lies to the left of the screen;
  ✓ transverse scan: patient's *right side* lies to the left of the screen.
✓ Use more gel if in doubt.
✓ If you are having difficulty obtaining or interpreting an image, consider the three Ps:
  ✓ Probe: orientation, gain, gel.
  ✓ Patient: genuine pathology, acoustic shadowing (e.g. ribs), bowel gas (US passes poorly through air), obesity.
  ✓ Physics: mirror artefact, reverberation.

Summary

- B-mode US is the type most commonly used in the ED.
- Higher frequency linear probes are used for more superficial scans and lower frequency curvilinear or phased array transducers for greater depth.
- US gel is used between the probe and the patient.
- Different tissues have different appearances; for example, bone cortex appears white and water appears black.
- On the image the patient's skin is at the top of the screen, and deeper structures towards the bottom of the screen.
- Longitudinal scan: patient's *head* lies to the left of the screen.
- Transverse scan: patient's *right side* lies to the left of the screen.
- Image artefact can be confusing or obscure anatomy, but can be helpful in some cases.

3

Abdominal aorta

Justin Bowra

The question: is there an abdominal aortic aneurysm?

The abdominal aorta passes from the diaphragm (surface anatomy: xiphoid process) distally through the retroperitoneum until its bifurcation into the common iliac arteries (approximately at the level of the fourth lumbar vertebra; surface anatomy: approximately at umbilicus) (Fig. 3.1). The aorta narrows as it descends. In adults its normal anteroposterior (AP) diameter is less than 2 cm. Although an oversimplification, a simple rule of thumb holds that a dilatation of the aorta 3 cm or more (i.e. 1.5× normal) is known as an *abdominal aortic aneurysm* (AAA). AAA may be fusiform or saccular. Most occur below the renal arteries.

Simplified approach to abdominal aorta AP diameter (Fig. 3.2):

- ≤2 cm   normal
- 2–3 cm   dilated but not aneurysmal
- ≥3 cm   aneurysm.

The larger the aneurysm the faster it dilates (LaPlace's Law) and the greater its risk of rupture. The risk of rupture is small if the diameter is less than 5 cm.

The elective operative mortality is approximately 5%. However, the mortality of ruptured AAA is 50% *provided the patient reaches the operating theatre (OT).*

Why use ultrasound?

Physical examination is unreliable in making the diagnosis. Alternative imaging techniques such as computed tomography (CT) take time to organize and require the transfer of an unstable patient out of the emergency department (ED). Bedside ultrasound (US) is rapid, safe, sensitive (97–100%) and allows ongoing resuscitation of the patient in the ED. Doppler imaging adds little and is not required.

Clinical picture

The clinical picture and its variability will be familiar to the experienced clinician.

- *The patient*: usually male (10× more common) and older than 50 years.
- *Pain*: usually severe abdominal pain, which may radiate to the back.

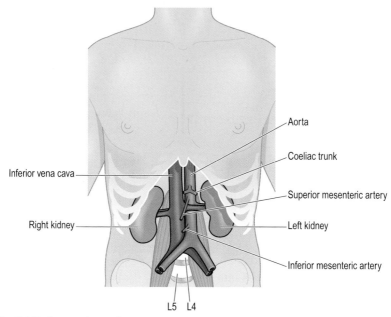

Fig. 3.1 Surface anatomy of aorta.

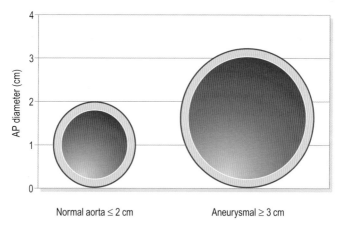

Fig. 3.2 Comparison of diameters of normal and aneurysmal aorta.

- *Shock*: not always present (e.g. contained rupture).
- *Abdominal mass*: above the umbilicus. Its absence does not rule out AAA.

- *Distal pulses*: usually normal.
- *Other presentations* are rare; for example, mass effect (such as bowel obstruction), torrential gastrointestinal bleeding from aortoenteric fistula.

- *Broad differential diagnosis*: for example, perforated viscus, peptic ulcer disease, acute coronary syndromes.

 If in doubt, assume the patient has AAA until proven otherwise.

Before you scan

- Move the patient to the resuscitation area.
- Address ABCs (NB: Aggressive fluid resuscitation of AAA may be detrimental. The optimum systolic blood pressure (BP) is probably 90–100 mmHg.)
- Get help: the doctor performing the scan should not also be resuscitating the patient.

 ED investigations (including US) and treatment must not delay urgent transfer of a shocked patient with suspected AAA to operation.

The technique and views

Patient's position

- Dictated by clinical picture.
- Supine is most practical.

Probe and scanner settings

- Curved probe: standard 2.5–3.5 MHz frequency is ideal.
- Standard B-mode setting.
- Focus depth 10 cm.
- Depth setting 15–20 cm.

Probe placement and landmarks

1. Start just below xiphisternum. Transverse position with probe marker to patient's right (Fig. 3.3).

2. Identify landmarks: vertebral body (VB; confirm bone's acoustic shadow) directly behind aorta, liver anterior and to the right, bowel (Fig. 3.4).

3. It is essential to identify and differentiate the *two* major vessels: inferior vena cava (IVC) and aorta (Table 3.1). The IVC is parallel and to the right and may be misidentified as the aorta, particularly in longitudinal section. Transmitted pulsation in the IVC can be misleading. If in doubt, use colour or pulse wave Doppler (see Figs 3.9 and 3.10).

4. It is helpful to identify some of the other vessels, especially the superior mesenteric artery (SMA) which runs parallel to the aorta and is easily recognized, surrounded by bright investing fascia (see Figs 3.1, 3.4, 3.6, 3.9 and 3.10). The origin of the SMA is a useful 'surrogate' for the level of the renal arteries, which are harder to see on US. For example, if an AAA is seen only below the origin of the SMA, then it is infrarenal.

5. Alter the depth setting, focus depth and gain to obtain the best image.

Fig. 3.3 Initial probe placement: transverse subxiphoid, probe directed posteriorly and probe marker to patient's right.

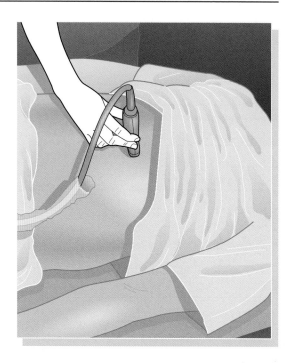

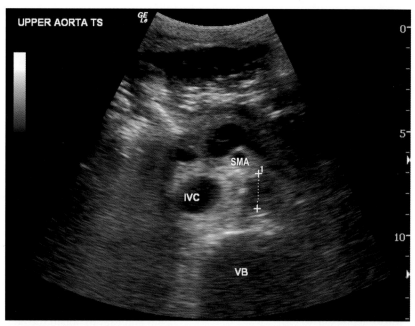

Fig. 3.4 Normal transverse view aorta, IVC, superior mesenteric artery (SMA) and vertebral body (VB). Aorta diameter measured.

Table 3.1 Identification of the major blood vessels

IVC	Aorta
To the anatomical right (*left* on screen)	To the left
Compressible (unless distal obstruction, e.g. massive PE)	Non-compressible
Thinner walls	Thick-walled, calcified
Oval cross-section	Round cross-section
	Smaller unless AAA

AAA = abdominal aortic aneurysm; PE = pulmonary embolism.

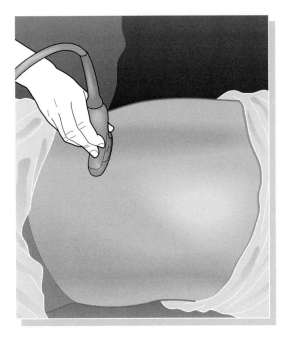

Fig. 3.5 Probe placement for distal transverse view of aorta.

6. Measure diameter from outer to outer wall. On transverse view, diameter may be obtained in either AP or horizontal direction, although the latter is probably more accurate. Save image.

7. Maintain the transverse position and sweep distally until bifurcation (Fig. 3.5). Measure diameter, save image.

8. Move the probe to longitudinal position and scan. Attempt to obtain a view of the aorta with origin of coeliac trunk or SMA (Fig. 3.6). Measure the AP diameter and save image.

9. Finally, scan the bladder (see Ch. 7, *Renal tract*). When severe, the pain of urinary retention can fool an inexperienced operator.

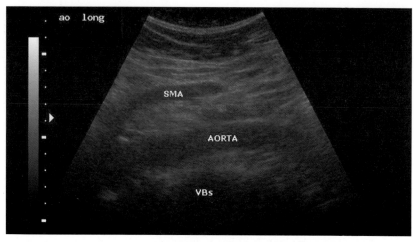

Fig. 3.6 Normal aorta longitudinal view (below) with origin of SMA and VBs.

Essential views

To rule out AAA, the aorta should be visualized in its entirety and a minimum of three hard copy images should be obtained:

- upper transverse section (Fig. 3.4)
- lower transverse section
- longitudinal section (ideally with origin of coeliac trunk or SMA) (Fig. 3.6).

All three views must include measurement of diameter.

 You have not ruled out AAA unless you can visualize the entire length of the aorta.

Handy hints

✓ Even for a skilled operator, sometimes bowel gas may render an image inadequate. If bowel gas is in the way, continue direct pressure with the probe on the abdominal wall (if pain permits) to displace the bowel. Altering the angle of the transducer may also help.

✓ Obese patients may be very difficult. Try the following to improve your image:

   ✓ Increase the image depth and alter the focus.

   ✓ Decrease the probe frequency.

   ✓ Decrease greyscale/increase contrast (refer to your machine's user manual).

   ✓ Scan through other windows; for example, from the right upper quadrant scanning through the liver will usually reveal the upper abdominal aorta.

✓ Measure diameter between the *outer* margins of each wall, not inner: this may overestimate the diameter but will avoid false negatives due to mural thrombus (Fig. 3.7).

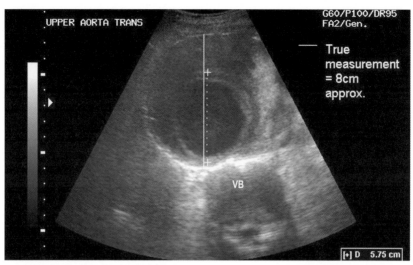

Fig. 3.7 Abdominal aortic aneurysm with mural thrombus, transverse section. Two anteroposterior (AP) measurements: the measurement between 'inner walls' underestimates the AP diameter. VB = vertebral body.

✓ The aorta may be ecstatic, and this will make measurement of diameter difficult. However, attempt to measure the diameter perpendicularly (Fig. 3.8); avoid taking a slice at an angle as this will overestimate the diameter.

✓ Doppler, either colour (Fig. 3.9) or pulse wave (Fig. 3.10), can help you differentiate between the aorta and the IVC.

✓ If on the first or second view you demonstrate AAA in an unstable patient, your priority is to transfer the patient to OT. Further views are not needed and waste time.

What US can tell you

• Is there an aneurysm (AAA)? US can detect AAA in at least 97% of cases, depending on operator and patient factors (e.g. obesity).

• Is there an aortic dissection? If a dissection extends to the abdominal aorta, its characteristic appearance of a mobile 'flap' will be seen (Figs 3.11 and 3.12).

What US can't tell you

• Can I *exclude* a dissection? Many aortic dissections will not extend into the abdominal aorta, and the sensitivity of US for dissection is low (5%). So if you suspect dissection, arrange another study (e.g. CT).

• Is the aneurysm leaking? US is insensitive in detection of retroperitoneal blood. If you detect AAA in a shocked patient, *assume* it has ruptured or is leaking.

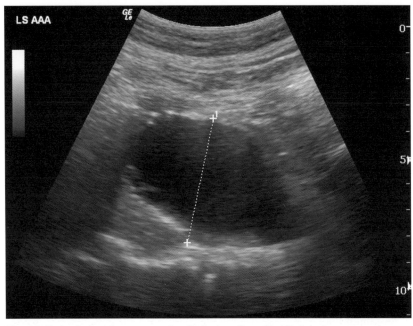

Fig. 3.8 Abdominal aortic aneurysm longitudinal section with AP diameter measured perpendicular to the aorta.

Fig. 3.9 Colour Doppler demonstrating flow in AAA and SMA.

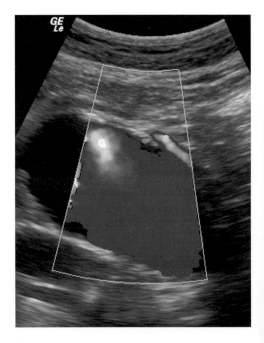

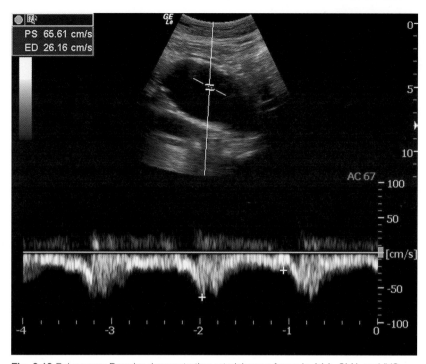

Fig. 3.10 Pulse wave Doppler demonstrating arterial wave forms in AAA. SMA and IVC also seen.

- Other causes of the pain (see above caveat regarding urinary retention). The differential diagnosis of severe epigastric pain in an unstable patient is broad. None of these differentials can be diagnosed or ruled out accurately by emergency US.

Now what?

- Unstable patient and AAA: notify surgical team immediately. The patient must be transferred immediately to OT or interventional suite for AAA repair.

- Unstable patient, unable to rule out AAA: this is a complex situation. Ongoing resuscitation, urgent surgical review and decision to proceed to OT (or further imaging such as CT) must be based on clinical likelihood of AAA.
- AAA ruled out by US: look for other cause of presentation (see above).
- Stable patient and AAA (or unable to rule out AAA): discuss with vascular surgeon. Patient requires further assessment and imaging (e.g. CT) to assess extent, renal artery involvement, etc.

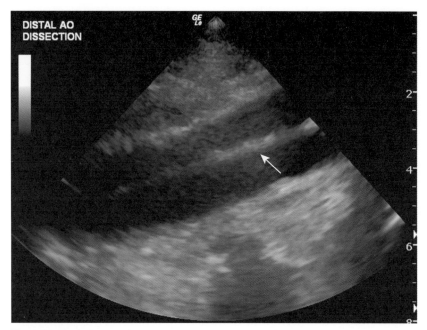

Fig. 3.11 'Flap' of aortic dissection (longitudinal).

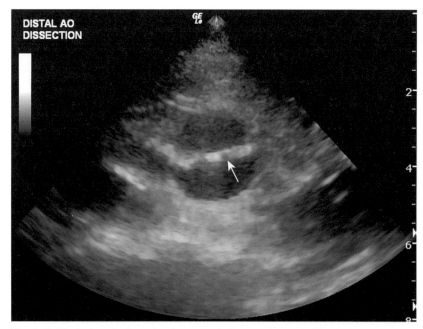

Fig. 3.12 'Flap' of aortic dissection (transverse). Same patient as in Fig. 3.11.

Summary

➡ Bedside US for suspected AAA is rapid, safe, sensitive and allows ongoing resuscitation of the patient in the ED.

➡ However, US and other ED investigations *must not delay* urgent transfer of a shocked patient with suspected AAA to OT.

➡ If in doubt, assume the patient has AAA.

➡ If you detect AAA in a shocked patient, *assume* it has ruptured or is leaking.

➡ You have not ruled out AAA unless you can visualize the entire length of the aorta.

➡ To rule out AAA, a minimum of three views should be obtained: upper and lower transverse sections and a longitudinal section. All three views must include measurement of diameter.

4

Focused assessment with sonography in trauma (FAST) and extended FAST (EFAST)

Russell McLaughlin

The question: is there free fluid?

Focused assessment with sonography in trauma (FAST) is a means of detecting free intraperitoneal fluid in the traumatized abdomen. Using Advanced Trauma Life Support (ATLS®) principles, the FAST scan is used as an adjunct to the primary survey assessment of circulation. It relies on the principle that free fluid (FF) such as blood collects in certain anatomical sites in the supine patient.

In the thorax, FF may be found in one of two potential spaces: the pericardium and pleural space. Pericardial blood, particularly if it collects rapidly, will progressively impair right ventricular diastolic filling until tamponade occurs. In a supine patient with a haemothorax, blood initially collects at the posterior lung bases. Like pericardial tamponade, massive haemothorax is a life-threatening condition that requires immediate drainage. Lung bases should routinely be included in FAST views. In addition to the lung bases, the upper anterior chest can be

visualized to detect the presence of pneumothorax. Adding these views is commonly known as extended FAST (EFAST). For details see Ch. 5, *Lung and thorax*.

In the supine abdomen, the most dependent potential spaces are scanned by FAST. Morison's pouch is found between the liver and right kidney. FF will collect here first. The lienorenal interface is the analogous potential space between the spleen and left kidney. Fluid on the left side will collect here or above the spleen (subphrenic fluid). In the pelvis, FF will collect in the pouch of Douglas (rectovesical pouch in the male) behind the bladder.

Why use ultrasound?

- Traumatic cardiac tamponade, tension pneumothorax and massive haemothorax may be rapidly fatal if not detected and treated in the emergency department (ED).
- Physical examination is unreliable for detection of cardiac tamponade in the ED setting, and is only 50–60% sensitive for detecting

significant intra-abdominal injury following blunt trauma.

- FAST is non-invasive, rapid, repeatable and can be performed at the bedside.
- FAST has supplanted diagnostic peritoneal lavage (DPL) as a reliable and non-invasive means of detecting abdominal FF in trauma patients.
- FAST is up to 90% sensitive and up to 99% specific for traumatic haemoperitoneum. (See 'Cautions and contraindications' below.)
- EFAST is more reliable than supine chest X-ray (CXR) in the detection of pneumothorax.
- US can be used to guide emergent pericardiocentesis and intercostal catheter placement.
- The use of contrast-enhanced ultrasound in trauma is beyond the scope of this chapter.

Clinical picture

- The patient will have suffered a form of trauma in which cardiac tamponade, intrathoracic or intraperitoneal bleeding is a possibility.
- FAST also plays a role in women in first trimester of pregnancy with abdominal pain, shock or per vaginal bleeding. In these patients, the presence of FF in the peritoneum suggests an ectopic pregnancy. For details, see Ch. 9, *Early pregnancy*.

Cautions and contraindications

- The only absolute contraindications to performing a FAST scan are the presence of a more pressing problem (such as airway obstruction) or a clear indication for emergency laparotomy (in which case FAST is not indicated).
- FAST is indicated only if it will affect patient management. For example, in the stable patient with blunt abdominal trauma, a negative FAST gives no information about solid organs or hollow viscus injury. Such patients may require other imaging such as computed tomography (CT).
- *Children.* Although CT scanning remains the investigation of choice in paediatric abdominal trauma, FAST does not expose children to radiation. The threshold for operative intervention in paediatric blunt abdominal trauma is higher than for adults.
- *Timing.* A very early scan may be falsely negative as sufficient intra-abdominal blood may not have collected in the dependent areas. Furthermore, occasionally a late scan may be falsely negative as clotted blood is of similar echogenicity to liver and may not be easily identified in Morison's pouch.
- *Operator.* The accuracy of FAST is operator-dependent, and the inexperienced scanner should be particularly wary of ruling out FF.

Urgent surgical consultation is mandatory in the unstable trauma patient suspected of having intra-abdominal injury.

FAST is indicated only if it will affect patient management.

FAST is not indicated in patients with a clear indication for immediate laparotomy; for example, penetrating injury in an unstable patient.

Before you scan

- Move the patient to the resuscitation area and assemble trauma team.
- Primary survey and resuscitation according to ATLS principles.
- The doctor performing the scan should not also be resuscitating the patient.

Technique and views

Patient's position

The patient should be in the supine position with arms abducted slightly or above the head to allow visualization of Morison's pouch and the spleen. Alternatively, the patient may be asked to fold their arms across their chest. This manoeuvre will be determined by the patient's conscious level and the presence of any upper extremity injury.

Probe and scanner settings

A low-frequency (4–7 MHz) probe should be used with the depth set according to the patient's body habitus.

The five views (Fig. 4.1)

1. *Pericardium.* The most common view used in this situation is the subxiphoid view. The probe is laid almost flat on the patient's epigastrium and angled towards the head. Advance the probe towards the xiphisternum. Apply enough pressure to allow the probe to indent the epigastrium, thus placing the probe deeper than the xiphisternum and costal margin (Fig. 4.2). Then sweep the probe in a left-to-right axis until the pulsation of the myocardium is visualized. The view obtained utilizes the liver as an acoustic window (see Ch. 2, *How ultrasound works*) and should demonstrate the four chambers of the heart (Fig. 4.3). Pericardial fluid appears as a black stripe (Fig. 4.4). In true cardiac tamponade the right ventricle will collapse during diastole. However, this can be difficult to assess for the non-echocardiographer, so clinical likelihood of tamponade must be taken into consideration when acting on a positive scan. In some patients, particularly the obese, it may be difficult to obtain clear subxiphoid images.

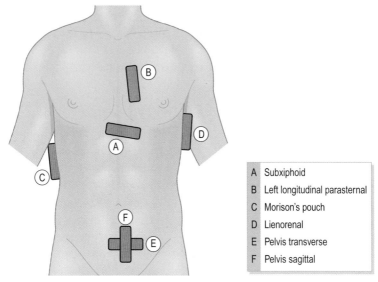

A	Subxiphoid
B	Left longitudinal parasternal
C	Morison's pouch
D	Lienorenal
E	Pelvis transverse
F	Pelvis sagittal

Fig. 4.1 Windows used for the FAST examination.

Fig. 4.2 Probe in subxiphoid pericardial position.

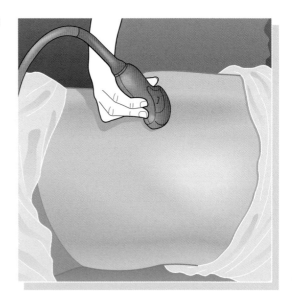

Two alternative pericardial windows are the parasternal long axis (PLAX; Fig. 4.5) and apical views. It is a good idea to practise these alternatives, as in some patients the subxiphoid window is inadequate. See Ch. 6, *Focused echocardiography and volume assessment.*

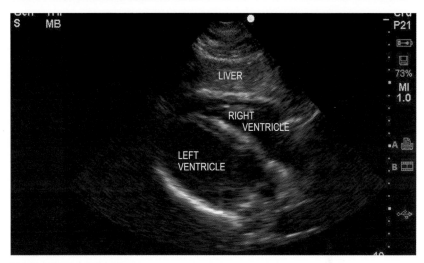

Fig. 4.3 Normal pericardium.

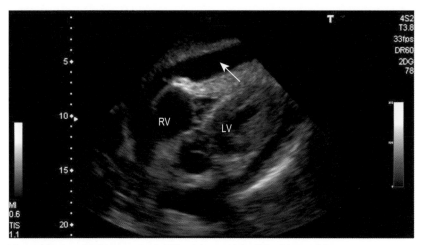

Fig. 4.4 Pericardial fluid (arrowed). RV = right ventricle; LV = left ventricle.

2. *Morison's pouch and right lung base.* Probe perpendicular to the line of the ribs and between the ribs where the costal margin meets the mid-axillary line on the right of the patient (Fig. 4.6). The view obtained utilizes the liver as an acoustic window and should demonstrate right kidney, liver, diaphragm (highly echogenic) and right lung base for pneumo/haemothorax (Fig. 4.7). Sweep the probe anteroposteriorly and alter the probe angle until you obtain a clear view of Morison's pouch.

Fig. 4.5 Probe in left longitudinal parasternal position.

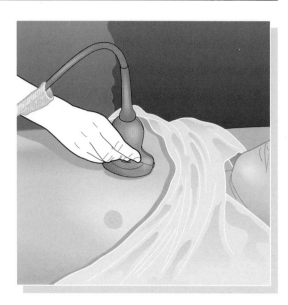

Fig. 4.6 Probe in Morison's pouch position.

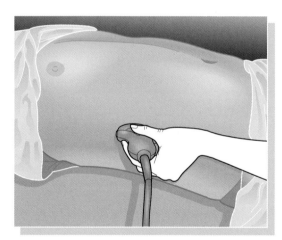

Unless clotted, FF appears as a black stripe in Morison's pouch (Fig. 4.8). Ask the patient to take a deep breath if possible, particularly if rib shadows obscure the area of interest; a clearer view of the liver and Morison's pouch is often obtained with this method.

3. *Lienorenal interface and left lung base*. Probe is angled on the left side as if looking for Morison's pouch but higher (ribs 9–11) and more posteriorly, in the posterior axillary line (Fig. 4.9). The spleen may be higher than expected and is more difficult to visualize than the liver. In a co-operative

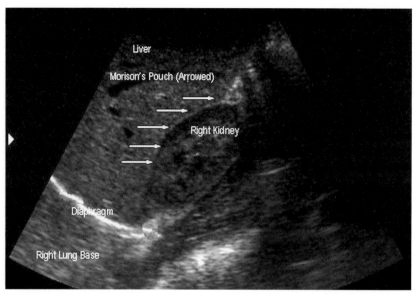

Fig. 4.7 Normal Morison's pouch.

patient, a deep breath may help. Sweep the probe and alter its angle as above, until you obtain a clear view of left kidney, spleen, diaphragm and left lung base (Fig. 4.10). FF will appear as a black stripe in the lienorenal interface (Fig. 4.11) or between the spleen and the diaphragm (subphrenic FF).

4. *Thorax.* Scan along the most and least dependent areas of both lungs to exclude haemothorax and pneumothorax respectively (see Ch. 5, *Lung and thorax*).

5. *Pelvis: sagittal and transverse.* For both pelvic views the fluid-filled bladder is utilized as an acoustic window. It is therefore important that the patient has a full bladder during this part of the examination. Ideally scan before catheterizing the patient. Otherwise, depending on urgency, clamp the indwelling catheter and allow the bladder to fill or fill the bladder with normal saline via the catheter.

To obtain the *sagittal* view, place the probe in the midline just above the pubis and angle it caudally at 45 degrees into the pelvis (Fig. 4.12). The view obtained should demonstrate a coronal section of the bladder and pelvic organs (Fig. 4.13). FF will be around the bladder or behind it (pouch of Douglas) (Fig. 4.14). In women the pouch of Douglas is deep to the uterus, so ensure that you scan deep enough to identify the uterus as

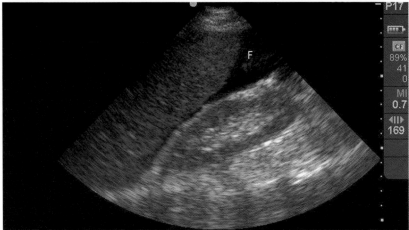

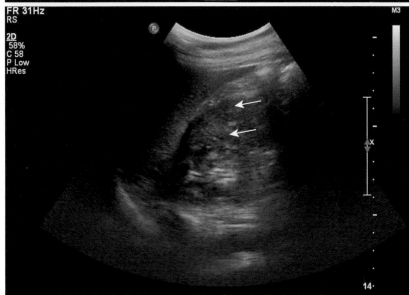

Fig. 4.8 (A) Free fluid (F) in Morison's pouch. (B) Clotted blood (arrowed) in Morison's pouch.

well as bladder. Ideally visualize the pelvic bones to ensure an adequate scan.

The *transverse* view is obtained by rotating the probe through 90 degrees from the sagittal position while maintaining contact with the abdominal wall (Fig. 4.15). Angle the probe into the pelvis, identify the bladder in transverse section and sweep the probe to visualize the pouch of Douglas and pelvic organs as above (Fig. 4.16).

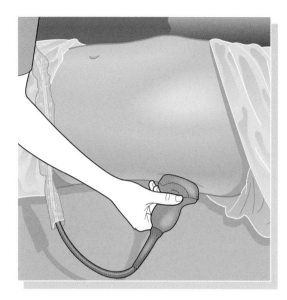

Fig. 4.9 Probe in lienorenal position.

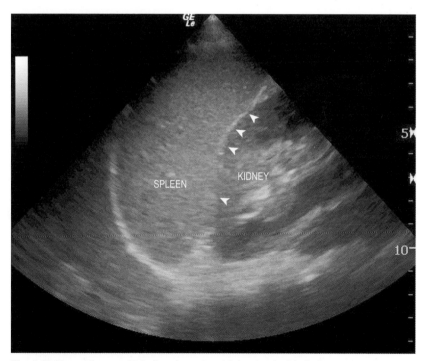

Fig. 4.10 Normal lienorenal interface (arrowheads), landmarks labelled.

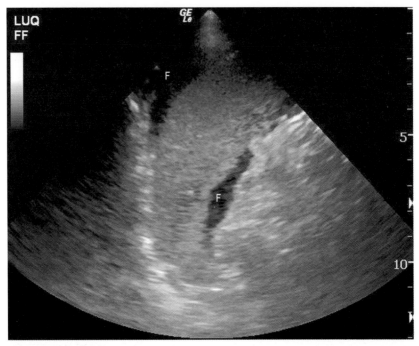

Fig. 4.11 Free fluid (F) in the lienorenal interface and subphrenic space.

Fig. 4.12 Probe in the sagittal pelvis position.

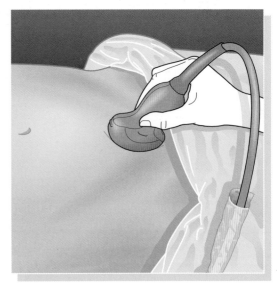

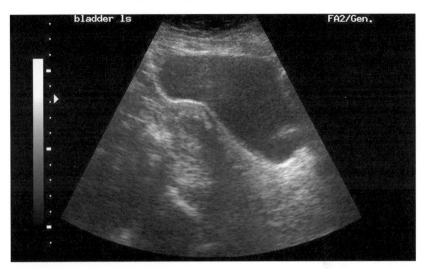

Fig. 4.13 Sagittal view normal pelvis.

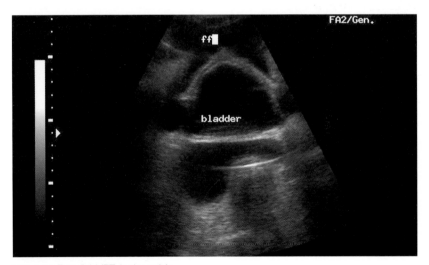

Fig. 4.14 Free fluid (FF) in the pelvis.

Extra views

Some authors recommend paracolic views. These probably do not add to the sensitivity of FAST and are not routine.

Essential views

To rule out FF, a minimum of five images should be obtained:

1. pericardium
2. Morison's pouch

Fig. 4.15 Probe in transverse pelvis position.

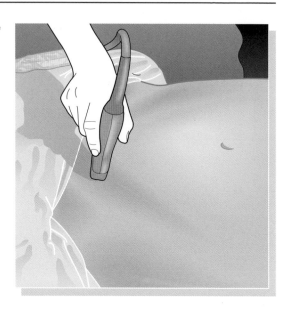

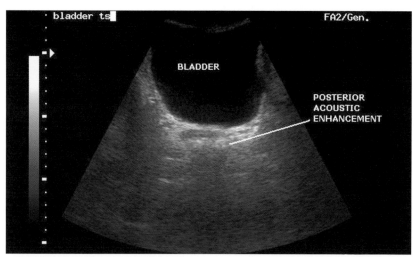

Fig. 4.16 Transverse view normal pelvis.

3. lienorenal interface
4. pelvic sagittal
5. pelvic transverse.

In addition, save cineloop or M-mode images of left and right pleural spaces.

Handy hints

✓ PLAX provides an alternative view of the pericardium.

✓ The lienorenal interface is more posterior and more cranial than you think!

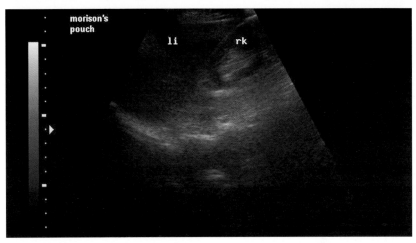

Fig. 4.17 Morison's pouch: inadequate view. li = liver; rk = right kidney.

✓ Scan through the respiratory cycle to minimize the effects of rib shadowing.

✓ If available, a probe with a small footprint can scan between ribs.

✓ If you still find it difficult to obtain clear views of Morison's pouch (Fig. 4.17) or the lienorenal space, slide the probe superiorly until you view the highly echogenic diaphragm. Use this as the landmark to identify the adjacent pleural space and liver/spleen.

✓ Beware false-negative scans. In the presence of small amounts of FF, a single view of Morison's pouch or lienorenal interface may be falsely negative. Hence, scan through a number of planes to rule out FF. If you still suspect FF, consider serial scans or other investigations.

✓ Also note that free blood is not always black (echo-poor). If clotted, it may be the same density as the liver and/or kidney.

✓ Similarly, scan any positive findings of FF through a number of planes and observe for peristalsis, pulsation and displacement with respiration. This allows FF to be differentiated from false positives due to fluid-filled structures such as inferior vena cava, gall bladder and intraluminal bowel fluid.

✓ Other causes of false-positive scans include:

  ✓ Fat (e.g. pericardial fat pad).

  ✓ Ascites.

  ✓ Mirror artefact (see below).

✓ Fluid in the bladder is required to visualize the pelvis.

✓ If FF in the pelvis cannot be distinguished from mirror artefact (see Ch. 2) then scan the pelvis through a number of planes; only FF should persist. Alternatively, the bladder can be partially emptied. Mirror artefact 'shrinks' with the emptying bladder while FF remains constant.

✓ Repeat the scan, particularly if a stable patient becomes unstable.

✓ If, on the first or second view, you demonstrate FF in an unstable patient, further views are not needed and waste time.

What FAST can tell you

FAST can determine the presence of the following:

- free intraperitoneal fluid
- pericardial fluid
- pleural fluid.

What FAST can't tell you

FAST cannot determine the following:

- source of FF
- nature of FF; for example, blood versus ascites
- presence of solid organ or hollow viscus injury
- presence of retroperitoneal injury.

Now what?

Urgent surgical consultation is mandatory in the unstable trauma patient with suspected intra-abdominal injury.

FAST is not indicated in patients with a clear indication for immediate laparotomy; for example, penetrating injury in an unstable patient.

- Unstable patient and pericardial fluid: suspect cardiac tamponade. Prepare for emergent pericardiocentesis.
- Unstable patient and pleural FF: suspect massive haemothorax. Emergent intercostal catheter drainage.
- Unstable patient and intra-abdominal FF: immediate transfer to OT for laparotomy.
- Unstable patient, inadequate or negative scan: ongoing resuscitation, clinical reassessment for other cause of instability, consider other investigation (e.g. CT, DPL) or exploratory laparotomy. While still in ED, frequent re-scanning for subsequent fluid accumulation.
- Stable patient and negative scan: although FF is excluded, assess patient for solid organ and hollow viscus injury as well as extra-abdominal injuries.
- Stable patient and positive scan: abdominal CT.

Summary

➡ FAST is useful when assessing the traumatized abdomen and chest.
➡ FAST is indicated only if it will affect patient management.
➡ It does not replace sound clinical judgement.
➡ It must be used in conjunction with ATLS principles.

5

Lung and thorax

Justin Bowra, Paul Atkinson

How can lung ultrasound help me?

While it may seem counterintuitive to use ultrasound (US) in the thorax (as air scatters and reflects US waves), predictable findings and patterns can be used for diagnosis of thoracic pathology, and US can help to make invasive chest procedures safer. Lung US is a comparatively recent addition to emergency US. Its systematic use was first described by Lichtenstein in his textbook *General ultrasound in the critically ill* (Springer, 2002). Since then, critical care doctors worldwide have taken it up for the following indications:

Diagnosis of
- pleural fluid
- pneumothorax (PTX)
- pulmonary oedema
- consolidation.

Procedural guidance for
- thoracocentesis
- intercostal catheter (ICC) placement.

When scanning the thorax, US waves can reach the lungs through the acoustic windows provided by the abdomen or the intercostal spaces.

US waves will penetrate the tissues until they encounter an interface with air, at which point they will be reflected and scattered.

The normal lung has a characteristic appearance described below. Changes in the normal amount of air, fluid and tissue alter this appearance in a predictable fashion, which permits US diagnosis of certain conditions. For example, in the presence of pleural fluid, US waves will penetrate further into the thorax, allowing the fluid and deeper structures to be visualized. In the case of PTX, US waves will not penetrate through the intrathoracic air.

Why use US?

- Common conditions such as PTX and massive haemothorax may be rapidly fatal if not detected and treated urgently in the emergency department (ED), or pre-hospital setting. Physical examination may be unreliable for detection of PTX, and for differentiating pulmonary oedema and pneumonia in the ED setting. While the plain chest X-ray (CXR) remains the initial investigation of choice for the diagnosis of such conditions in the emergency setting, the reliability of plain radiography, especially in the supine patient, can be overestimated at times.

- Lung US is easy to learn, non-invasive, rapid, repeatable and can be performed at the bedside. It is more sensitive and reliable than mobile CXR in the detection of pleural fluid: it can detect as little as 100 mL, with sensitivity >97% and specificity 99–100%. In expert hands, lung US has been described as 98% sensitive and 99% specific for PTX, and 85.7% sensitive and 98% specific for pulmonary oedema. However, its operator dependence means that it is less accurate in the hands of novice scanners.

- Lung US has been used to aid the diagnosis of pulmonary embolus (PE), but its sensitivity is only approximately 74%, and therefore it has not been widely adopted in this area.

- Invasive procedures such as emergency thoracocentesis and ICC placement have a significant morbidity and a notable mortality rate. Lung US improves the safety of these procedures and is now the standard of care.

Clinical picture

- In the breathless patient: is there a PTX, a pleural effusion and/or pulmonary oedema?

- In the shocked patient: is there a tension PTX? Have we given too much fluid?

- The multitrauma patient: is there a PTX or a haemothorax? See also Ch. 4, *FAST and EFAST.*

- Why has the breathless/shocked patient not responded to initial treatment?

Cautions and contraindications

- The only absolute contraindications to performing lung US are the presence of a more pressing problem (such as airway obstruction) or lack of adequate operator training.

- The accuracy of lung US is operator-dependent, and the inexperienced scanner should be particularly wary of *ruling out* the conditions described.

 Lung US is very operator-dependent and is more reliable at ruling in conditions such as PTX than ruling them out.

Technique and views

Patient's position

This depends on the clinical picture. Ideally, as much as possible of the chest (front and back) should be scanned, but often this is impossible in the trauma or resuscitation setting.

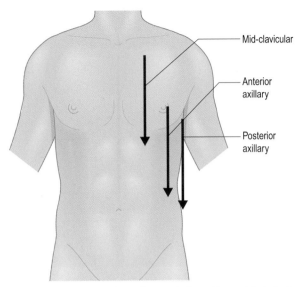

Fig. 5.1 Thorax scanning lines: posterior axillary, anterior axillary, mid-clavicular.

Probe and scanner settings

Theoretically the linear array (5–10 MHz transducer) should be used because of its high resolution, but often the phased array (cardiac) probe provides the best overall views of the lungs for determination of fluid, consolidation and fibrosis. Its small footprint is designed to use the intercostal spaces as acoustic windows.

Even a curved (abdominal) probe will suffice for an initial screen, and either the curved or phased array probe will already be active if proceeding from a cardiac or trauma scan.

The views

The key is to scan as much of the lung as possible, to avoid missing significant pathology. With that in mind, ensure that (at the very least) you scan along the anterior and posterior axillary lines, and along the anterior chest (mid-clavicular line). Scanning the least dependent (anterior) part of the chest will pick up a small PTX, and the most dependent (posterior/inferior) part will pick up small pleural fluid collections (Fig. 5.1).

Although one may begin scanning anywhere in the chest, the novice should begin with a right upper quadrant view as for FAST (focused assessment with sonography in trauma; see Fig. 4.6). Align the probe in the long axis of the patient's body (coronal plane), with probe marker to the patient's head. First identify the liver and *diaphragm*. The diaphragm will appear as a curved echogenic (bright) line. The brightness of the diaphragm is in part due to the reflective interface it provides with

45

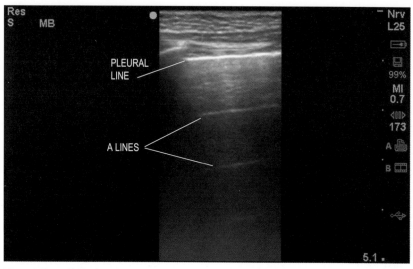

Fig. 5.2 Normal thorax with depth at 5 cm, and A lines, US image.

air-filled lung behind it (remember, US waves are scattered and reflected at the first air interface they encounter). Next slide the probe up to the thorax. Reduce image depth to 5–10 cm depending on body habitus, and reduce focal zone depth to about 2–3 cm. Keep the probe at right angles to the ribs initially to allow you to use the rib shadows as a landmark (later you'll change the probe to parallel to maximize your view of B lines).

Identify the ribs by the shadows they cast, then look between and below the ribs for the highly echogenic pleural line (Fig. 5.2).

What to look for

Normal lung

- As US waves enter the chest, they pass though skin, subcutaneous tissue, intercostal muscles and then arrive at the pleura. As the pleural surfaces are apposed, waves penetrate to the visceral pleura (which lies on air-filled lung tissue) where they are then reflected.

- *Normal pleura.* The normal pleural line resembles a 'sparkling curtain' sliding back and forth as the patient breathes. (The sparkle represents scatter from the air in the lung.) This is known as *dynamic sliding* and its *absence* is the most reliable US sign of PTX.

- *A lines.* These are reverberation artefacts from the pleural line. They are horizontal and static and represent *normal reverberation artefact* from the pleura (Fig. 5.2).

- *B lines.* These are hyperechoic reverberation effects from air/water interfaces in the interlobular septa. They can be considered the

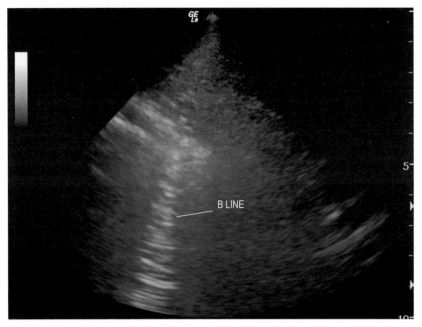

Fig. 5.3 B line, US image.

ultrasonic equivalent of Kerley B lines. They are vertical and move with respiration. Also called 'comet tails', they are bright, thick vertical lines which reach to edge of screen and obliterate A lines (Fig. 5.3). Up to one-third of normal subjects have B lines in dependent regions, but if they are widespread they are termed *lung rockets* and are considered pathological (see below).

• Z lines are also vertical, but unlike B lines these fade quickly, don't obliterate A lines and have no apparent significance (Fig. 5.4).

PTX

• In PTX, the pleural surfaces are separated by air, and waves are now reflected at the interface of the parietal pleura with the air of the PTX itself. Therefore, movement of the visceral pleura and lung deep to the PTX cannot be seen, leading to loss of the typical appearances outlined above (Fig. 5.5).

• *Absence of dynamic sliding* (see above) is a key feature of PTX on US. However, it can be found in a number of other conditions as well:
  • the lung apices
  • chronic airflow limitation
  • right main stem intubation (absence of sliding on the left side)
  • pleural tethering (e.g. due to lung cancer at the periphery) (Fig. 5.6).

• More specific to PTX is the *lung point sign* (Fig. 5.7). This window

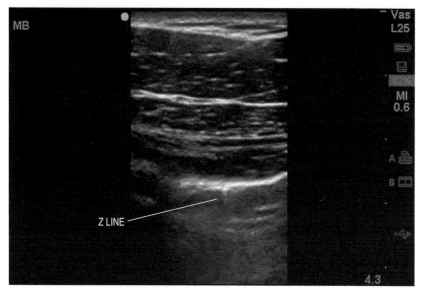

Fig. 5.4 Z line, US image.

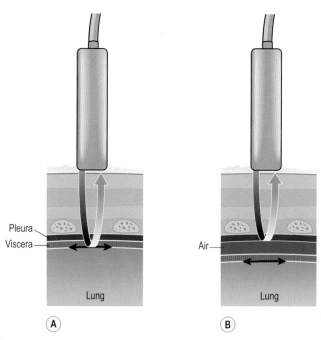

Fig. 5.5 Explanation of lung sliding and its absence in pneumothorax.

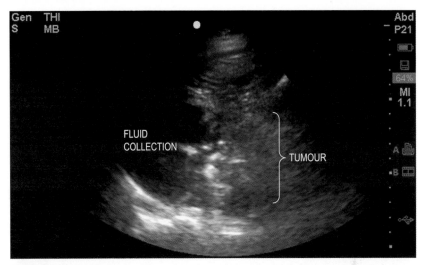

Fig. 5.6 Pleural tethering from lung carcinoma, US image. Heterogeneous tumour (partly liquefied).

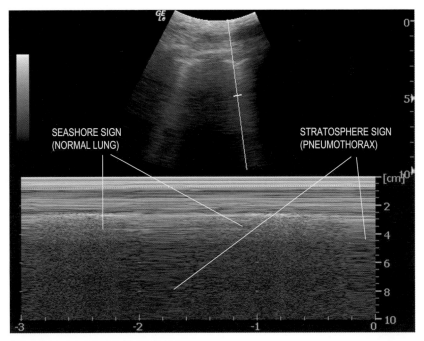

Fig. 5.7 Lung point sign, M-mode image.

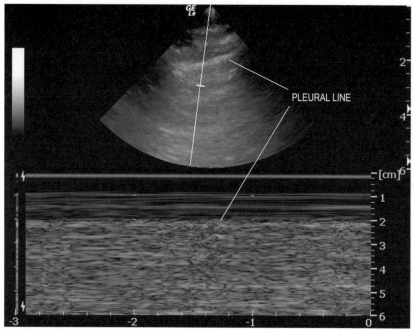

Fig. 5.8 Seashore sign (normal lung), M-mode image.

represents the site where normal lung gives way to PTX, so that on one side of the image sliding is present, while on the other side it is absent. Some say this is the only truly reliable sign of PTX. However, it can also be seen in cases of pleural tethering.

 If you can see dynamic sliding, there is no PTX at that site. (But there may be a PTX elsewhere in the lung field.)

 If you can't see dynamic sliding, there *may* be a PTX at that site.

 If you see the lung point sign, there is *probably* a PTX at that site.

- M-mode is not essential but sometimes helps confirm the presence/absence of dynamic sliding. In M-mode, normal dynamic sliding is described as the *seashore sign* (Fig. 5.8) whereas the absence of normal sliding is described as the *stratosphere sign* (Fig. 5.9).

Pleural fluid

- If present, this is found in the most dependent regions of the thorax. Its appearance varies from black/anechoic (fresh blood, transudate/exudate) to grey/echogenic (e.g. clotted blood, exudate). If fluid is present in the costophrenic angle, US waves will be transmitted through it allowing visualization of

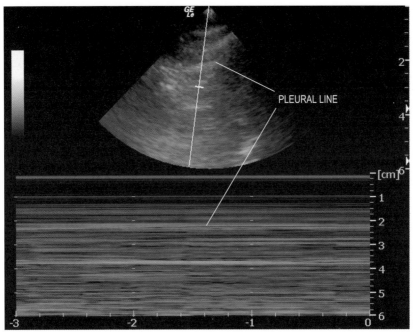

PLEURAL LINE

Fig. 5.9 Stratosphere sign (pneumothorax), M-mode image.

diaphragm and liver/spleen (which in the normal lung 'disappear' with inspiration) (Fig. 5.10; see also Fig. 2.1). Also note that in the presence of pleural fluid, the diaphragm is less echogenic as it is no longer forming an interface with reflective air-filled lung.

Lung rockets

- 'When several B lines are visible in a single scan, the pattern evokes a rocket at lift-off, and we have adopted the term *lung rockets*' (Lichtenstein, 2002, p. 106) (Fig. 5.11). Occasional rockets can be normal (see note above), but if widespread, bilateral, and three or more per window, these are pathological.

- Pathological lung rockets are found in the following disease states (described collectively by Lichtenstein as the *alveolar-interstitial syndrome*):
  - pulmonary oedema
  - widespread pneumonia
  - chronic interstitial diseases; for example, fibrosis.

 The three features of pathological lung rockets:
- bilateral (present in both lung fields)
- widespread (present in several lung windows)
- at least three per window.

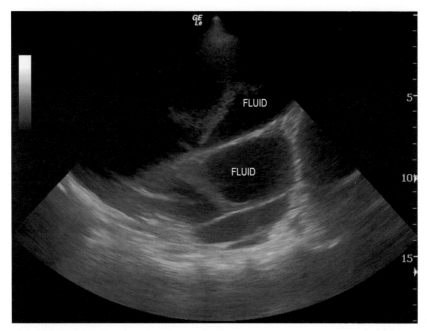

Fig. 5.10 Multiloculated pleural effusion, US image.

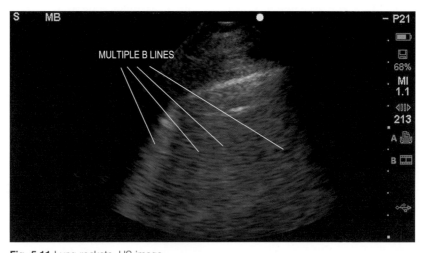

Fig. 5.11 Lung rockets, US image.

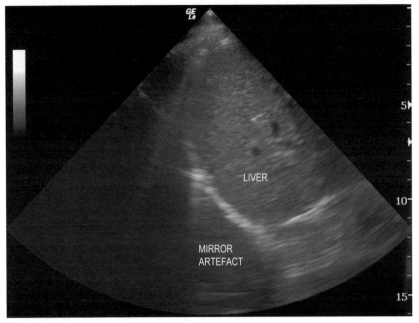

Fig. 5.12 Mirror artefact from liver, US image.

- The presence of lung rockets can be used to guide fluid resuscitation and diuresis. For example, when rockets start to appear during aggressive intravenous fluid resuscitation, one should slow down or cease fluids.

Alveolar consolidation

- If you can see the structural anatomy of lung tissue, then it is abnormal. Put simply, non-aerated lung resembles the tissue of solid organs such as the liver. This can occur in several disease states: notably collapse, consolidation, contusion, atelectasis and malignancy (Fig. 5.6).

- Note, however, that at the lung bases the presence of apparent consolidation is most often simply due to mirror artefact (Fig. 5.12) (see also Ch. 2, *How ultrasound works*).

- If the area of consolidation extends to the pleura, you will visualize it on US. However, US cannot be used to rule out consolidation, as it cannot pick up areas of consolidation deep to normal lung tissue (the air-filled lung scatters and reflects US waves).

 Lung US can sometimes rule in consolidation, but it cannot rule it out.

Handy hints and pitfalls

✓ Start with a low-frequency (phased array or curved) probe to help you identify anatomical structures such as the *diaphragm*. Carefully orientate yourself to structures lying above and below the diaphragm.

✓ Switch to the linear probe to examine the pleura in more detail.

✓ Identify the ribs then turn the probe parallel to them—the pleura lies just deep to the level of the ribs.

✓ Hold the probe still—look for pleural sliding for a period of time before moving to the next window.

✓ Scan as much of the lung fields as possible, or you will miss small PTX and fluid collections.

✓ Lung sliding can be absent in a number of conditions (see above), but if the lung point is identified, this points towards a diagnosis of PTX. Rarely a lung point will be seen at a point of pleural tethering.

✓ Mirror artefacts can resemble basal consolidation and are more common (see Ch. 2, *How ultrasound works*). If you cannot distinguish consolidation from mirror artefact, scan the area of interest through a number of windows.

✓ It can be difficult to differentiate fluid in the left hemithorax from pericardial fluid when scanning the heart. Pericardial fluid passes in front of the descending aorta, while pleural fluid surrounds the descending aorta.

✓ Similarly, peritoneal fluid can be mistaken for pleural fluid. The key is to carefully identify the diaphragm. Pleural collections are superior to the diaphragm, and the lung can be seen 'floating' in large collections.

✓ Not all vertical lines are B lines. Z lines can resemble B lines, and pseudo-rockets can be seen in subcutaneous emphysema (they do not move with respiration, and there are no normal rib shadows above them).

✓ Not all rockets infer the presence of pulmonary fluid. They can also be seen with widespread pneumonia and widespread fibrosis. Rockets can also be normal in lowest intercostal space, and similarly posterior lung rockets can be normal in supine patients (in dependent lung).

✓ Because the patient's fluid status changes with treatment, repeat the scan frequently, particularly if a stable patient becomes unstable.

✓ When choosing a site for thoracocentesis, remember the following simple points to minimize the chance of inadvertent needle placement in the abdomen (see also Ch. 10, *Ultrasound-guided procedures*).

✓ Begin with a curved or phased array probe to help you identify the anatomy, before changing to a high-frequency linear probe.

✓ Scan through the entire respiratory cycle, and ask patient to take maximal inspiration and expiration.

✓ Scan in two planes.

✓ Scan with the patient in the same position you'll insert ICC and carefully identify an insertion point away from underlying organs.

✓ Finally, use real time US for the procedure if at all possible.

What lung US can help tell you

• The breathless patient: is there a PTX, a pleural effusion and/or pulmonary oedema?

• The shocked patient: what is the volume status? (Use in conjunction with US assessment of inferior vena cava (IVC) diameter, the heart and abdomen.)

• The multitrauma patient: is there a PTX or a haemothorax? (See also Ch. 4, *FAST and EFAST*.)

• Why has the breathless/shocked patient not responded to initial treatment?

• Where shall I place the thoracocentesis needle or ICC? (See also Ch. 10, *Ultrasound-guided procedures*.)

• Sometimes lung US can identify PE, but that is outside the scope of this chapter (see comment in 'Why use Ultrasound').

What lung US can't tell you

• You cannot determine the nature of pleural fluid: for example, fresh blood versus transudate.

• You cannot rule out alveolar consolidation.

• You cannot rule out a tiny PTX or effusion.

 If you want to find all pneumothoraces, perform a CT scan.

Now what?

• Negative CXR but US shows PTX, in a stable patient: consider CT.

• Negative CXR but US shows PTX, in an unstable patient: treat PTX.

• Negative CXR but US shows PTX, stable patient but rushing to operating theatre (OT)/helicopter: consider ICC.

• Unstable patient and large pleural fluid: suspect massive haemothorax. Emergency ICC.

• Widespread lung crepitations in a breathless patient, plus lung rockets and large IVC (see Ch. 6, *Focused echocardiography and volume assessment*): suspect pulmonary oedema.

• Widespread lung crepitations in a breathless patient, but no lung rockets and normal calibre IVC: pulmonary oedema unlikely. Search for other causes (e.g. pneumonia).

• Aspirating a PTX, no further air forthcoming but still *absent* pleural sliding in superior chest: reposition catheter and continue aspiration.

• Aspirating a PTX, no further air forthcoming and pleural sliding *present* in superior chest: aspiration is complete.

Summary

➡ Lung US is useful when assessing the breathless patient.

➡ In combination with cardiac/IVC US (see Ch. 6, *Focused echocardiography and volume assessment*), lung US assists in the diagnosis of pulmonary oedema and guides fluid management.

➡ It does not replace sound clinical judgement.

6 Focused echocardiography and volume assessment

Justin Bowra, Robert Reardon, Conn Russell

Why use ultrasound?

Basic echocardiography is a rapid, goal-directed cardiac study performed in the critical care setting. Unlike formal echocardiography, it aims to provide a qualitative assessment of overall cardiac function rather than answer specific questions such as presence of valvular lesions. When combined with assessment of other body areas, such as the inferior vena cava (IVC), abdominal aorta (Ch. 3), lung (Ch. 5), and leg veins for deep venous thrombosis (Ch. 12), it can assist in diagnosis and guide management.

In this chapter, echocardiography and IVC assessment will be discussed, followed by a suggested ultrasound (US) algorithm in the patient with undifferentiated shock.

Focused versus comprehensive echo

The skills required to perform and interpret a comprehensive echo exam can only be acquired with extensive formal training under expert supervision. This training is outside the practical achievement of most doctors

in the emergency department (ED) or intensive care unit (ICU). It has been shown, however, that a rapid goal-directed, focused study can be carried out with a limited amount of training. The focused exam comprises simple two-dimensional (2D) images, without any of the more complex quantitative measurements carried out during a comprehensive exam. Focused echo has the added advantage that the clinician carrying out the exam is also treating the patient, and thus is best placed to relate the echo findings to the clinical situation.

Transthoracic versus transoesophageal echocardiography

It can be difficult to obtain good-quality images with transthoracic echo on acutely ill patients for a variety of reasons (e.g. position, ambient lighting, pain, mechanical ventilation). For this reason, transoesophageal echo is often favoured for a full quantitative study in the critically ill patient. It has been shown, however, that images sufficient for a limited study are possible by the transthoracic route in up to 97% of patients. Transoesophageal echo also requires further equipment and training outside the scope of this text.

Classic haemodynamic patterns

Haemodynamically unstable patients often present with classic patterns seen on focused echo.

These patterns become more obvious as the clinical condition deteriorates, and are often easily seen with focused imaging.

- Poorly contracting left ventricle (LV): cardiogenic shock.
- Dilated right ventricle (RV), underfilled LV: massive pulmonary embolus (PE).
- Pericardial fluid with RV collapse: tamponade.
- Vigorously contracting, underfilled LV (with small end systolic and end diastolic diameter): hypovolaemia.
- Vigorously contracting, underfilled LV (with small end systolic and normal end diastolic diameter): septic shock.

The differences between hypovolaemia and sepsis may be subtle, but initial treatment with fluid loading will be similar for both groups.

Diagnosis

Focused echo and volume assessment can help answer the following questions:

- Why is the patient shocked?
- Is there pericardial fluid or tamponade?
- Is there a massive PE?

- Are the ventricles contracting normally?
- Are the cardiac chambers dilated?
- Does the patient need intravenous fluid, inotropes or pressors?
- Are there any other obvious abnormalities?

Time is of the essence in commencing resuscitation and establishing a diagnosis in the shocked or arrested patient. US assists in determining the patient's intravascular status, and is faster, safer and easier than alternatives such as invasive central venous pressure (CVP) monitoring.

Intervention

- US guides ongoing fluid management.
- US can be used to guide emergent pericardiocentesis in cardiac tamponade.
- US-guided central venous cannulation (CVC) access: for CVP monitoring and delivery of fluids and inotropes.

It should be remembered that the techniques described below are no substitute for formal echocardiography. If an advanced echocardiogram is required, arrange a formal study. However, the phased array probes and software available on most modern portable US machines will allow you to visualize the heart and pericardium sufficiently to answer the basic questions listed in this chapter.

 If an advanced echocardiogram is required, arrange a formal study.

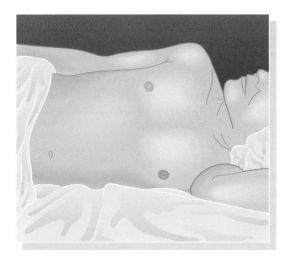

Fig. 6.1 Patient in left lateral position.

Scanning the patient

Preparation

- Move the patient to the resuscitation area, attach monitors and oxygen, and address ABCs.
- Get help: the doctor performing the scan should not also be resuscitating the patient.
- Arrested patient: arrest team and protocols as per local practice.
- Sterile, dedicated equipment is ideal if performing US-guided intervention such as pericardiocentesis, but this must be balanced against the urgency of the situation.

 ED investigations (including US) must not delay resuscitation of a shocked or arrested patient.

Patient's position

- Dictated by clinical picture (e.g. arrested patient).
- Supine is most practical.

- Cardiac scan: ideal patient position is left lateral (Fig. 6.1), which brings the heart to the left of the sternum (hence less shadowing) and closer to the probe. However, adequate scanning is still possible in supine or semi-recumbent position.

Probe and scanner settings

- Probe: phased array or microconvex probe (small footprint minimizes rib artefact).
- Preset: cardiac preset differs from abdominal preset in several ways. The most obvious is that the image is inverted, which can pose a challenge to the novice sonologist. For example, on parasternal long axis (PLAX) view (see below), the apex of the heart points to the left of the screen, not the right. (If it is difficult to interpret the images, then you can use the machine's controls to invert the image back to 'normal'.) Less obvious is that the

image is less 'jerky' (higher frame rate for better visualization of motion) and the image is more 'black and white' (decreased dynamic range) on cardiac preset. This is to aid in performing measurements of cardiac chambers.

- If a cardiac probe and preset are unavailable, use a standard curved low-frequency probe on abdominal preset. The images will be sub-optimal but should suffice for some of the basic questions (particularly the presence of cardiac standstill and pericardial tamponade).

- Most modern ED US machines also have Doppler and M-mode capability. This will assist in transthoracic scans of the heart and pericardium.

- For further tips, see 'Handy hints and pitfalls' below.

Cardiac scan
Normal anatomy

The LV is seen deep to the RV on a parasternal or subcostal view and is much thicker-walled. The relative strength and wall thickness of the LV usually give it a convex shape on US and cause it to push forward into the thinner-walled RV (see Figs 6.5 and 6.6).

Using the views described below, echocardiographers view and describe the heart in planes (Fig. 6.2):

1. Long-axis view: this runs parallel to the heart's long axis. In the parasternal position (with probe marker pointing to patient's right shoulder) this allows simultaneous visualization of the LV and the outflow tract of the RV (Figs 6.3A and 6.4).

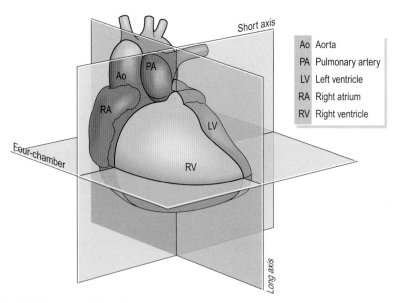

Ao	Aorta
PA	Pulmonary artery
LV	Left ventricle
RA	Right atrium
RV	Right ventricle

Fig. 6.2 The echocardiographic axes.

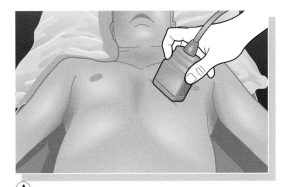

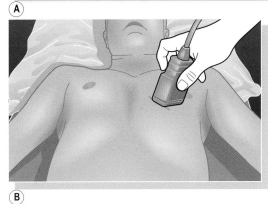

Fig. 6.3 Probe in left parasternal position.
(A) Long-axis orientation.
(B) Short-axis orientation.

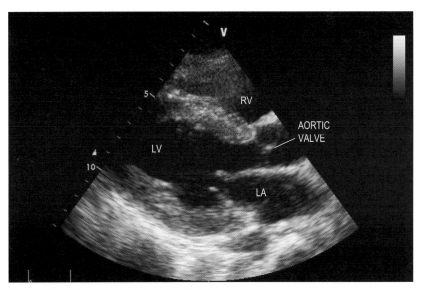

Fig. 6.4 Normal parasternal long axis, US image.

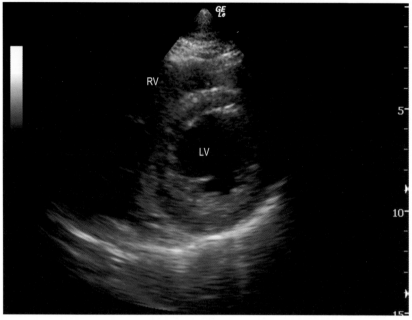

Fig. 6.5 Normal parasternal short axis, US image.

2. Short-axis view: perpendicular to the long axis (probe marker pointing to left shoulder in the parasternal position) (Figs 6.3B and 6.5). Sliding the probe (maintained in this position) along the long axis will allow a series of 'sectional' views of the LV and RV, which allows an assessment of relative wall thickness and contractility (Fig. 6.6).

3. Four-chamber view: the long-axis view which simultaneously demonstrates all four chambers. This is usually obtained from the apical window (see below) but may be obtained from the subcostal window.

It is important to note that these planes are not longitudinal or transverse with respect to the patient, as the heart itself is obliquely angled. While this may seem obvious, it represents a departure from the longitudinal and transverse windows described in this and other texts of emergency US.

Normal chamber sizes/wall thickness in the average adult are as follows:

- LV diameter (diastole) 3.5–5.7 cm (4–6)

- RV diameter (diastole) 0.9–2.6 cm (1–3)

- RV diameter $<0.6 \times$ LV

- LV wall and IV septum <1.1 cm

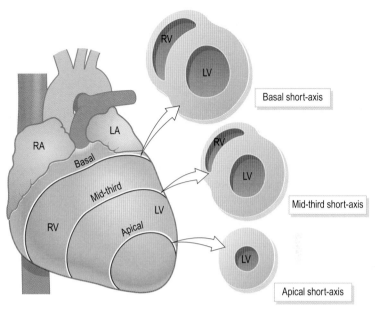

Fig. 6.6 Series of short-axis views of the heart.

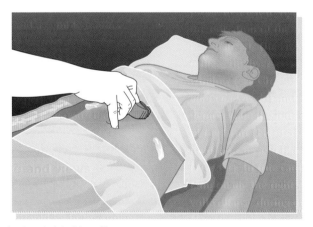

Fig. 6.7 Probe in subxiphoid position.

- RV wall <0.5 cm
- Left atrium (LA) diameter and aorta root each <4 cm.

Windows

Several windows (probe positions) are used. The following are useful for the critical care sonologist (see also Ch. 4, *FAST and EFAST*):

- Subcostal/subxiphoid, with the probe angled superiorly into the thorax. This window uses the liver as a sonographic window (Figs 6.7 and 6.8). It is the standard window

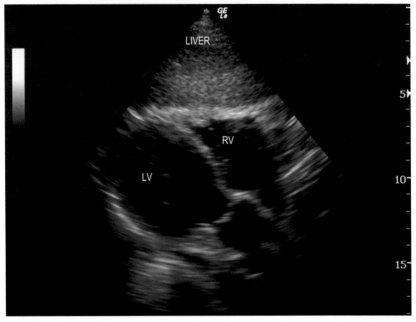

Fig. 6.8 Normal subcostal/subxiphoid, US image. Note that this image is backwards from the standard subcostal orientation.

taught in FAST, and may be the only available during cardiopulmonary resuscitation (CPR) or in ventilated patients.

- Left PLAX. Note that this is in the long axis to the heart, not the patient. Align the probe with the marker to the patient's right shoulder (Figs 6.3A and 6.4). Using caliper measurement of the LV and M-mode scanning, this view affords a rough estimation of LV function (see below).

- Left parasternal short axis: in the same position as PLAX but rotated 90 degrees clockwise so that the probe marker is towards the left shoulder (Figs 6.3B and 6.5). This view is the best for assessing regional wall motion.

- Apical four-chamber: probe placed at the apex beat and angled towards the right scapula, with the probe marker in the 3 o'clock position (directed at the patient's left arm) (Figs 6.9 and 6.10).

While any window may suffice for identification of pericardial fluid or cardiac standstill, a combination is required to visualize the heart more fully (e.g. to comment on LV motion). Sliding the probe down from the parasternal and across to the apical window will also assist in complete visualization.

Several other 'windows' have been described and include right parasternal and suprasternal. These are beyond the scope of this chapter.

Assess the following in particular:

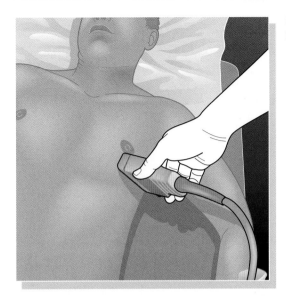

Fig. 6.9 Probe in apical position.

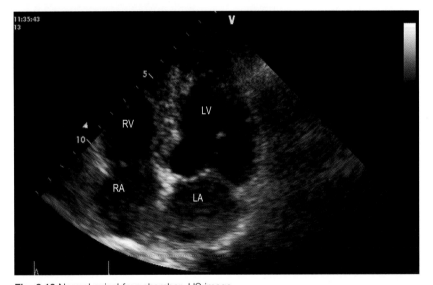

Fig. 6.10 Normal apical four chamber, US image.

- pericardium
- LV size: too small/too big/just right
- LV contractility: a lot/a little/just right
- RV size
- RV contractility.

Pericardium

Pericardial fluid most commonly appears as a black stripe around the heart (Fig. 6.11; see also Fig. 4.4). However, its appearance is determined by its nature; for example,

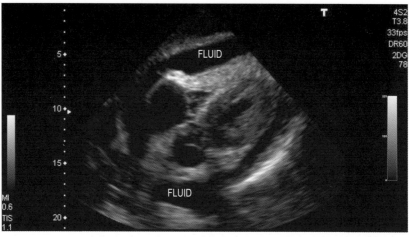

Fig. 6.11 Pericardial fluid, US image.

clotted blood will demonstrate a density similar to that of soft tissue.

As noted in Ch. 4, in true cardiac tamponade the pressure of the tamponade on the RV impairs RV filling during diastole and the RV collapses (Fig. 6.12). However, this can be difficult to assess for the non-echocardiographer. Therefore, stick to the following guide:

- Fluid seen just in systole: a small effusion (probably physiological).
- Fluid also seen in diastole: likely to be a pathological effusion but still may be too small to cause symptoms (Fig. 6.11).
- Heart rocking within a large effusion: significant and usually requires pericardiocentesis. (NB: large pericardial effusions are often chronic, and may not lead to significant compromise.)
- Small right atrium and ventricle (RA and RV), which collapse and do not open up in diastole, plus

distended IVC: the most reliable US indicators of tamponade (Figs 6.12 and 6.15).

However, bear in mind that the diagnosis of tamponade is a clinical one, so the above findings must be interpreted in the light of the clinical picture.

False-positive findings of pericardial fluid may be seen in the presence of pleural fluid or an anterior fat pad. A fat pad will often have a stippled appearance, and will move along with the heart.

False negatives may occur in the presence of localized or loculated pericardial effusions, which may be missed by US. Hence, scan cautiously and through as many views as possible (see below) to rule out false positives and negatives.

LV size

- If the *entire* LV is dilated and contracting poorly, consider causes

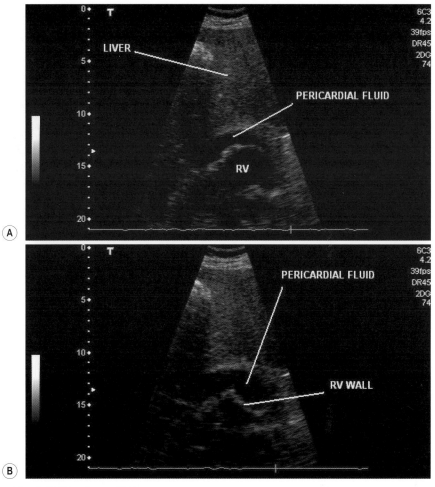

Fig. 6.12 RV collapse, US image.

of global hypokinesis (cardiomy-opathy) such as viral, idiopathic and alcoholic cardiomyopathy or severe sepsis (Fig. 6.13).

- If the LV chamber size is small and the walls meet in systole, consider hypovolaemia or LV hypertrophy.

LV contractility

- Cardiac standstill. In the arrested patient with PEA (pulseless electrical activity) asystole, this carries an extremely poor prognosis.
- LV hypokinesis. Global hypokinesis is usually obvious but difficult for the novice, and focal abnormalities may be difficult to appreciate. If one wall is seen not to move inwards during systole then myocardial infarction may be the cause of the patient's picture (cardiogenic shock).

67

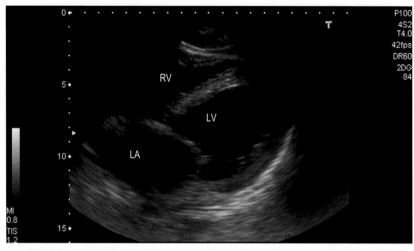

Fig. 6.13 Dilated LV, US image.

- Hyperkinetic heart. In the absence of arrhythmia or acute valve disease (particularly acute mitral regurgitation), cardiogenic shock is unlikely if the heart is beating strongly. Assess the patient for hypovolaemia or causes of high-output states such as anaemia and thyrotoxicosis.

RV size and contractility

The RV lies in front of the LV, appears smaller on US and has an irregular shape which conforms to the higher-pressure LV. Like the LV, the RV should contract forcefully during systole and fill during diastole. It is best to estimate RV size in comparison to LV, as absolute measurements may not be accurate (especially in PLAX).

- A small, hyperkinetic RV accompanying similar changes in the LV suggests hypovolaemia.

- A dilated RV which impinges on the LV suggests high pressures in the pulmonary circulation, either acute (e.g. massive PE) or chronic (e.g. cor pulmonale) (Fig. 6.14). In the latter condition, the RV wall should be thickened.

The RV is generally the only cardiac chamber able to dilate acutely. Dilation of other chambers indicates pre-existing cardiac disease.

Other obvious abnormalities

Other abnormalities (e.g. gross valve pathology) are often seen on echo, and may be of significance to the clinical presentation. While acting on this pathology is not encouraged, images can be stored for referral and review by an expert.

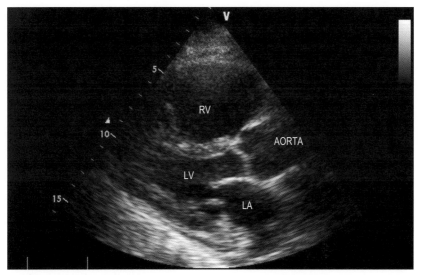

Fig. 6.14 Dilated RV which impinges on the LV (massive PE), US image.

Table 6.1 Guide to intravascular volume status

IVC diameter (cm)	Collapse with sniff	Interpretation	Estimated CVP (mmHg)
<1.5	>50%	Underfilled	0–5
1.5–2.5	>50%	A little dry	5–10
1.5–2.5	<50%	Euvolaemic	10–15
>2.5	<50%	Overload	>15

 Avoid attempting more than a rough description of ventricular appearance and function. Over-interpretation of poor-quality images is dangerous. Formal assessment is complex and requires calculations, equipment and experience not possessed by the average ED sonologist.

IVC: diameter and collapse

Theory

The normal IVC collapses with inspiration. Its cross-sectional area is greater than that of a normal aorta. IVC diameter and collapse with inspiration are used as a non-invasive surrogate for CVP measurement. The values given in Table 6.1 have been suggested as a guide to the patient's intravascular volume status. Like CVP measurement, this technique allows only a rough estimate of volume status. The values relate to stable patients with spontaneous respirations and may not apply to acutely ill patients and those with positive pressure ventilation.

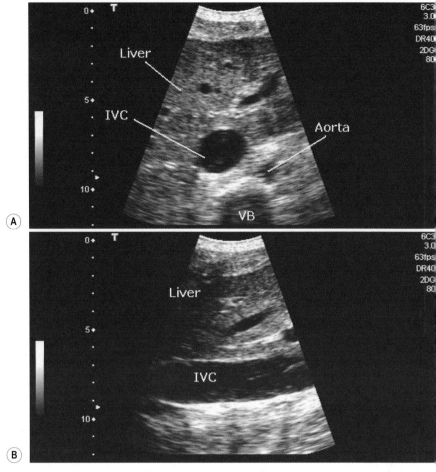

Fig. 6.15 Distended, non-compressible IVC, US image. VB = vertebral body.

- If IVC is distended, not collapsing with inspiration and not easily compressed by direct pressure with the US probe, in a shocked patient this strongly suggests distal obstruction (Figs 6.15 and 6.16). Potential causes include LV failure, massive PE, tension pneumothorax and cardiac tamponade. However, bear in mind that there are many other causes for elevated caval pressure such as pulmonary hypertension.

- Conversely, if IVC appears under-filled, this strongly suggests hypovolaemia as the cause of the patient's shock (Fig. 6.17).

Technique

- Patient position is crucial to the interpretation of IVC assessment. A moment's reflection is enough to

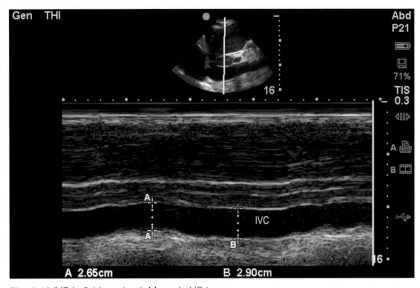

Fig. 6.16 IVC in fluid overload, M-mode US image.

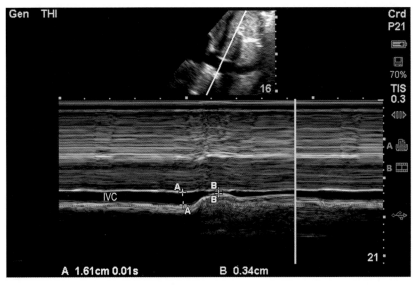

Fig. 6.17 Underfilled IVC, M-mode US image.

recall that IVC measurements will be lower in the left decubitus position than in the right decubitus. In practice, most patients will be supine or semi-recumbent because of their clinical condition.

- Either of two windows can be used: the subcostal or right upper quadrant (both of these views use the liver as a sonographic window). Whichever is used, be sure to scan the IVC in two planes: both long axis and transverse. For simplicity, only the subcostal approach is described here.

- Either the phased array (cardiac) or curved probe is suitable for IVC assessment.

- As for abdominal aortic aneurysm (AAA) scans (Ch. 3, *Abdominal aorta*), place the probe in the subxiphoid position, angled directly posteriorly (see Fig. 3.3). Identify landmarks and differentiate between the aorta and IVC as described in Chapter 3.

- Then angle the probe upwards, following the IVC as it traverses the diaphragm to enter the RA.

- Measure the IVC about 2–3 cm caudal to the hepatic vein inlet, not at the level of the diaphragm. Measure its maximal diameter (this will be in expiration) in two planes.

- Then measure the minimum IVC diameter using the sniff test: ask the patient to sniff quickly (this will cause intrathoracic pressure to fall rapidly, and a normal IVC will collapse).

- M-mode scanning can be used to capture maximum and minimum diameters on a single image (Figs 6.16 and 6.17).

Suggested US approach to the patient with undifferentiated shock

Although the patient with no clinically apparent cause for shock is uncommon, it is common to encounter the shocked patient with two or three equally plausible causes for his/her condition. With that in mind, many US algorithms have been proposed to help improve diagnostic certainty in the shocked patient. The following is a typical example. Clearly, not all windows will be required in every patient.

- Cardiovascular: heart (tamponade, LV/RV size and contractility), aorta (AAA), IVC (volume status).

- Thorax: pneumothorax, pleural effusion, pulmonary oedema, alveolar consolidation.

- Abdomen: free fluid, gall bladder.

- Leg veins: above knee deep vein thrombosis (DVT).

Handy hints and pitfalls

✓ Keep repeating the scan during ongoing resuscitation: trends are more important than single readings.

✓ Be aware of your own limitations: you are not a cardiologist! Avoid the temptation to comment on subtle or more complex pathology (such as valve disease) unless you have been trained formally in echocardiography.

✓ Beware of over-interpretation of echo images (e.g. diagnosing massive PE on the basis of a chronically dilated RV or IVC diameter in a patient with chronic pulmonary hypertension).

✓ Although RV changes may occur with conditions such as massive PE, even experienced echocardiographers find that the RV is difficult to assess. This is because of its irregular shape and acoustic shadowing from the overlying sternum.

✓ Images should be recorded for review and expert referral when appropriate.

✓ Any of the three cardiac windows described above may suffice for identification of pericardial fluid or cardiac standstill. However, no single window will yield adequate views in every patient, and a combination of views is required to visualize the heart adequately (e.g. to comment on LV motion).

✓ For example, in the obese, the subcostal window yields poor cardiac views, and the parasternal window may yield poor results in emphysematous patients. Hence, it is wise to practise the other views described above at every opportunity.

✓ If in doubt regarding your findings, continue treatment on clinical grounds and consider more definitive investigation; for example, formal urgent bedside echocardiogram.

✓ Tips to improve cardiac image quality:

  ✓ Decrease the gain (Ch. 2, *How ultrasound works*) and increase the contrast—this will sharpen the image.

  ✓ Most machines have cardiac presets—use them!

  ✓ Altering the probe frequency may help to reduce artefact due to cardiac wall motion

  ✓ In a ventilated patient, temporarily turning off the positive end-expiratory pressure (PEEP) may improve images from all windows.

Now what?

- Cardiac standstill in PEA or asystole: poor prognosis. Review decision to continue CPR.

- Pericardial fluid, clinical picture of tamponade: arrange urgent bedside echocardiography if possible. Prepare for pericardiocentesis.

- Small, hyperkinetic heart: suspect hypovolaemia. Continue fluid resuscitation and assess response.

- Gross LV hypokinesis: consider LV myocardial infarction or other causes of hypokinesis such as severe sepsis.

73

- IVC is distended and not easily compressible: suspect distal obstruction. Reassess patient for quickly reversible causes such as tension pneumothorax and cardiac tamponade. US may suggest PE but is inadequate for diagnosis, so if clinical picture suggests massive PE, decision to proceed to formal investigation (e.g. CT) or urgent thrombolysis depends on clinical picture.
- IVC underfilled: consider hypovolaemia. Continue fluid resuscitation and assess response.
- Unstable patient and AAA: notify surgical team immediately. The patient must be transferred immediately to operating theatre (OT) for AAA repair.
- Massive pleural fluid collection causing cardiorespiratory compromise, whether traumatic (haemothorax) or atraumatic (e.g. malignancy associated): urgent thoracocentesis via intercostal catheter.
- Unstable trauma patient and intra-abdominal free fluid (FF):

immediate transfer to OT for laparotomy.
- Inadequate scan: refer (e.g. for urgent echocardiogram) and continue resuscitation and treatment on clinical grounds.

 If in doubt about cardiac findings, refer to an echocardiographer.

Summary

➡ Bedside US in the shocked or arrested patient is rapid, safe and allows ongoing resuscitation of the patient in the ED.
➡ Bedside US assists rapid differentiation of many of the causes of shock but is not a substitute for formal echocardiography.
➡ US can assist urgent interventions in the shocked/arrested patient such as pericardiocentesis and central venous access.
➡ However, US and other ED investigations must not delay resuscitation.
➡ If in doubt, continue treatment on clinical grounds, and consider more definitive investigation: for example, urgent bedside echocardiogram.

7

Renal tract

Justin Bowra, Stella McGinn

Introduction

Ureteric colic, acute renal failure (ARF) and urinary retention are common emergency department presentations. The timely diagnosis of hydronephrosis in ureteric colic and ARF is valuable and may rapidly change management (e.g. prompting urgent decompression in pyonephrosis). Basic ultrasound (US) scanning of the kidneys and bladder is rapid, safe and relatively easy to learn, particularly for emergency physicians who are trained in focused assessment with sonography in trauma (FAST).

Why use US?
Five good reasons

1. ARF: US quickly determines whether this is post-renal (obstruction). This is a surgical emergency which requires intervention such as nephrostomy. For example, in bladder outlet obstruction, US will demonstrate a large bladder and bilateral hydronephrosis.

2. Pyonephrosis (pyelonephritis plus obstruction of that kidney). This is a surgical emergency which requires urgent nephrostomy.

3. US confirms the diagnosis of urinary retention.

4. US can be used to guide the safe placement of a suprapubic catheter (SPC) using the curved probe, or an infant bladder tap using the linear probe. (For details on SPC insertion, see Ch. 10, *Ultrasound-guided procedures*.)

5. Ureteric colic: Non-contrast abdominal CT of kidneys, ureters and bladder (CTKUB) is still the investigation of choice. Patients with ureteric colic often have sonographically normal kidneys and may even have ureteric jets. Therefore, focused US cannot be used to rule out a stone in the ureter. However, it can suggest its presence, and can rule out abdominal aortic aneurysm (AAA) as a differential diagnosis.

Avoid misdiagnosis of 'ureteric colic' in patients with more sinister pathology such as symptomatic abdominal aortic aneurysm (AAA).

Anatomy

- Normal adult kidneys measure approximately 10–12 cm × 5 cm × 3 cm. Their size increases with patient height, and *decreases* with age. Importantly, the left and right kidneys should be about the same size.

- Situated below the diaphragm, they lie obliquely in the retroperitoneum at the approximate level of vertebral bodies T12–L2. The right kidney lies more inferiorly than the left due to the bulk of the liver above (Fig. 7.1). Each kidney descends up to 2 cm in a full inspiration.

- The kidney is invested in a capsule (brightly echogenic on US) surrounded by dark perinephric fat, which in turn is surrounded by fascia. The kidney may be divided into the renal cortex and medulla (dark on US) which surrounds the echogenic renal sinus, which consists of the pelvicalyceal system, renal vessels and fat (Figs 7.2 and 7.3). The calyces unite in the renal pelvis, which is the funnel-shaped origin of the ureter.

- The bladder lies in the pelvis. As it fills it extends behind the symphysis pubis into the lower abdomen. A full bladder is dark (echo poor), well demarcated and demonstrates posterior acoustic enhancement. As it contracts, the normal wall

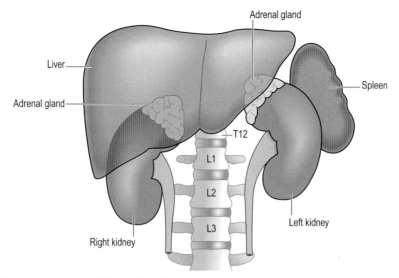

Fig. 7.1 Anatomical relations of the kidneys, anterior view.

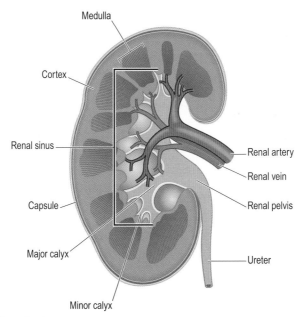

Fig. 7.2 Kidney structure.

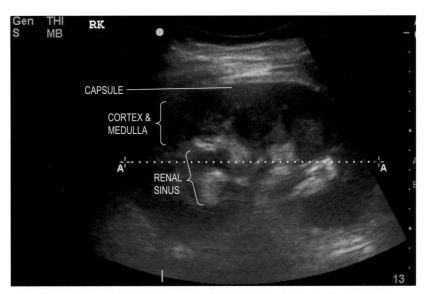

Fig. 7.3 Normal kidney longitudinal section, US image. Echogenic capsule, dark cortex and medulla, and bright renal sinus are indicated.

uniformly thickens. (If you see *localized* thickening, refer for a formal scan.)

What US can tell you

Is the bladder full?

Acute urinary retention is essentially a clinical diagnosis. However, clinical assessment of the bladder is difficult in some patients (e.g. the obese), and US can rapidly confirm the presence of a full bladder.

What size are the kidneys?

In renal failure, the kidneys' dimensions and appearance on US will assist in formulating a differential diagnosis. For example, large, cystic kidneys suggest familial polycystic kidney disease. Bilaterally small, scarred kidneys suggest chronic renal disease such as long-standing glomerulonephritis. Significant difference in size between the kidneys suggests renovascular disease or reflux nephropathy.

Is there hydronephrosis? (see Figs 7.7 and 7.8)

Hydronephrosis may be defined as dilatation of the renal pelvis and calyces due to obstructed outflow of urine. For a diagnosis of hydronephrosis, the minimum anteroposterior (AP) diameter of the renal pelvis has been defined variously as 10 mm, 17 mm and 20 mm. This threshold also changes with age and pregnancy. For this reason, many radiologists prefer not to set an absolute

threshold but to use a combination of findings (such as unilateral large kidney with renal pelvis and calyceal dilatation) to diagnose hydronephrosis.

Note that *calyceal dilatation* is also an important part of this definition, as the presence of pelvic dilatation with normal calyces may be found as a normal variant in patients with extrarenal pelvis.

Hydronephrosis is most commonly due to ureteric obstruction. Acute hydronephrosis is of most interest in the following clinical situations:

- Clinical suspicion of ureteric calculus (stone)
- ARF: to exclude post-renal cause.

False positives for hydronephrosis

- A full bladder can dilate both renal pelves.
- So can being pregnant.
- An extrarenal pelvis can look dilated but the calyces will be normal.
- Cysts: don't communicate with collecting system but this can be tricky to demonstrate.

False negatives for hydronephrosis

- Dehydrated patient.

Is the hydronephrosis acute or chronic?

Hydronephrosis is chronic if the renal cortex is thinned and the kidneys are scarred.

Is there pyelonephritis?

Pyelonephritis is a clinical diagnosis. Furthermore, in pyelonephritis, most

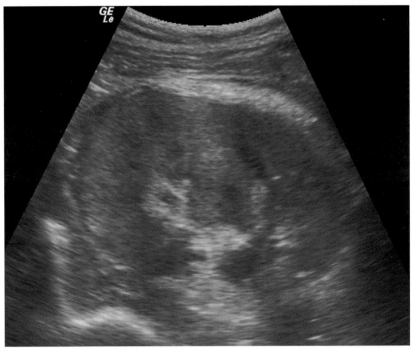

Fig. 7.4 Pyelonephritis with perinephric fluid, hypoechoic areas, loss of corticomedullary differentiation, US image.

kidneys appear normal on US. Therefore, US is not used to rule out this diagnosis.

However, US may sometimes rule it in, by demonstrating one or more of the following (Fig. 7.4):

- Enlarged kidney.
- Surrounding (perinephric) fluid: analogous to 'stranding' on CT.
- Altered echotexture: in parts hypoechoic (oedema, abscess) or hyperechoic (haemorrhage).
- Loss of corticomedullary differentiation.

- Absent perfusion in some areas (using Doppler).

Can I see a stone in the kidney or ureter?

On US a renal calculus is brightly echogenic and demonstrates posterior acoustic shadowing. A stone demonstrated in the renal pelvis (e.g. staghorn calculus) may be the cause of the patient's symptoms or incidental.

False positives for stones:
- calcified vessels.

False negatives for stones:
- stones too small to see with US.

Where can I safely place the SPC?

As discussed in Chapter 10 (*Ultrasound-guided procedures*), US ensures adequate placement of the SPC.

What US can't tell you

- It cannot *exclude* a stone in the ureter. US is unable to image the ureters as they descend towards the bladder. Therefore, it is poor at excluding ureteric calculi.
- It cannot determine the renal function. However, the presence of small scarred kidneys suggests chronic renal failure.

The technique and views

Patient position, probe and scanner settings are as for FAST (Ch. 4, *FAST and EFAST*) with the patient supine. The decubitus position may also be used (see below).

Probe placement and landmarks

1. *Right kidney.* Begin with probe parallel to the ribs where the costal margin meets the mid-axillary line on the right of the patient. Using the liver as an acoustic window, this view demonstrates right kidney, liver and highly echogenic diaphragm (see Fig. 4.7). The kidneys lie obliquely (with the upper poles more posterior than the lower poles), so alter the probe angle until you obtain a clear long-axis view of the kidney. Ask the patient to take a deep breath if rib shadows obscure the kidney, to obtain a clearer view. Alter depth, focus and gain until the kidney image fills the screen.

2. Measure the maximum length of the kidney from pole to pole (see Fig. 7.3).

3. Then rotate the probe to obtain a transverse or short-axis view and measure the dimensions (Fig. 7.5). For both axes, angle the probe back and forth to sweep the beam *past* each kidney to avoid surprises! This will ensure you don't miss pathology.

4. *Left kidney.* This view is harder to obtain, because the spleen is not as effective an acoustic window as the liver and the kidney is higher. Begin on the left side as if looking for Morison's pouch but higher (ribs 9–11) and more posteriorly, in the posterior axillary line (see Figs 4.9 & 4.10). Again, a deep breath may help. Sweep the probe and alter its angle as above, until you obtain a clear view of left kidney, then alter depth and focus to improve the image.

5. An alternative method of scanning the left kidney is to lie the patient in the right decubitus position and scan through the left costovertebral angle (Fig. 7.6).

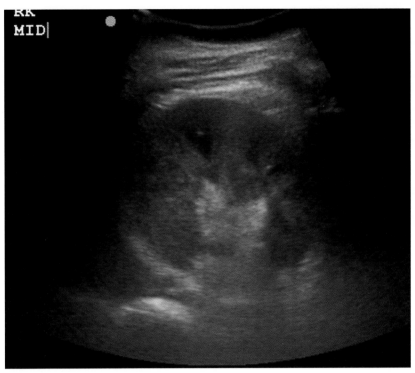

Fig. 7.5 Transverse section, US image, same kidney as in Fig. 7.3.

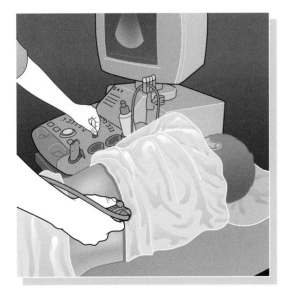

Fig. 7.6 Patient in right decubitus position, probe scanning for left kidney.

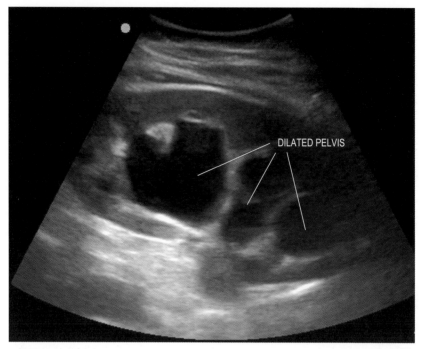

DILATED PELVIS

Fig. 7.7 Hydronephrosis, US image.

6. Another method is to place the probe in the right or left hypochondrium and direct it posteriorly. This view may be limited by bowel gas.

7. Hydronephrosis appears as a dark, echo-poor area in the pelvicalyceal system, communicating with the ureter (Fig. 7.7). Mild hydronephrosis may be subtle, but the presence of any dark, echo-poor areas within the normally bright renal sinus should raise the suspicion of hydronephrosis.

8. Measure the AP diameter of the renal pelvis and compare the two kidneys. If the diameter of one renal pelvis is greater than 10 mm, then hydronephrosis may be present (Fig. 7.8). (Note, however, that hydronephrosis may be bilateral.)

9. Assess the calyces. If they are also distended (Figs 7.7 and 7.8) then hydronephrosis is confirmed.

10. Cysts may mimic hydronephrosis. They are also echo-poor but are found in the cortex rather than the collecting system and do not communicate with the renal pelvis. Cysts are a common finding and may be benign or malignant. The presence of multiple cysts suggests polycystic kidney disease or age-related multicystic disease (Fig. 7.9).

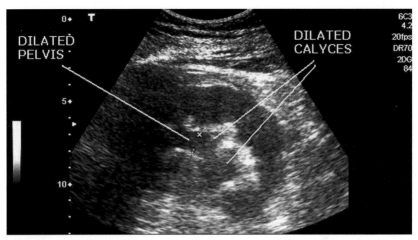

Fig. 7.8 Hydronephrosis, renal pelvis measured, US image.

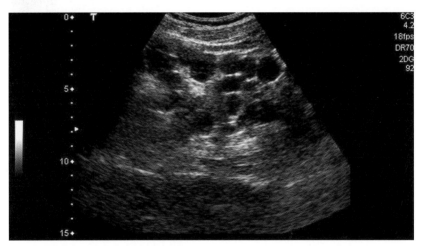

Fig. 7.9 Multiple renal cysts, US image.

11. When seen on US, calculi are brightly echogenic and demonstrate posterior acoustic shadowing.
12. *Bladder.* Scan as for FAST (Ch. 4, *FAST and EFAST*), with the probe angled into the pelvis. Be sure to scan in two planes, scanning right through and past the bladder from one side to the other to ensure full visualization of the bladder.
13. *Ureteric jets.* These are the normal 'jets' of urine that exit the ureters as the bladder gradually fills. In the ideal world, the presence of jets indicates patent ureter and rules out ureteric colic. But, in

the real world, low-grade obstruction can still occur in the presence of symmetrical jets. However, if no jet is observed on the affected side of a patient with suspected ureteric colic, this makes the diagnosis much more likely.

To scan for jets:

- Image the ureteric orifices
- Colour Doppler
- Watch each side carefully
- Can take >1 minute to see.

Handy hints and caveats

✓ Avoid misdiagnosis of 'ureteric colic' in patients with more sinister pathology such as symptomatic AAA (see Ch. 3, *Abdominal aorta*).

✓ The left kidney is more posterior and more cranial than you think!

✓ Scan through the respiratory cycle to minimize the effects of rib shadowing.

✓ If necessary, use a phased/sector probe to scan between ribs.

✓ If you still find it difficult to identify the kidneys, slide the probe proximally until you view the highly echogenic diaphragm. Use this as a landmark and slide the probe distally.

✓ If a kidney is still not visible or displays unusual features, consider congenital abnormalities such as absent or horseshoe kidney.

✓ Scanning a transplanted kidney (usually found in the iliac fossa) is usually easier as the kidney is more superficial than native kidneys.

✓ When measuring kidney dimensions, avoid underestimation of length, which is easily done if the US beam intersects the kidney obliquely or if both poles are not seen simultaneously (Fig. 7.10).

✓ Remember to compare the left and right kidneys (e.g. when assessing renal dimensions).

✓ Beware *false positives* and *false negatives* for hydronephrosis (see above).

✓ If the renal pelvis *and calyses* are dilated, then hydronephrosis is present.

Now what?

- Hydronephrosis in a patient with single kidney and ARF: urgent decompression (e.g. nephrostomy) by a radiologist or urologist.

- Clinical and US features of pyonephrosis also mandate urgent decompression.

- Clinical picture of ureteric colic plus hydronephrosis strongly suggests the presence of ureteric calculus. Assess for severity (e.g. mild versus gross hydronephrosis) and complications (such as infection and renal impairment) and discuss with a urologist.

- Clinical picture of ureteric colic, *no* hydronephrosis: arrange further imaging for ureteric calculus (e.g. non-contrast CT) as per local protocol.

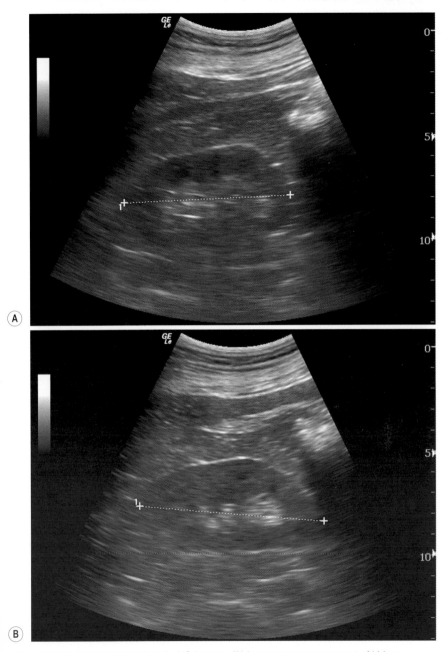

Fig. 7.10 Estimating kidney length, US images. (A) Inaccurate measurement of kidney length: plane of probe is oblique to long axis of kidney. (B) Same kidney, more accurate measurement, but upper pole not well visualized.

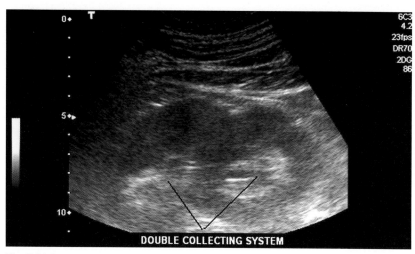

Fig. 7.11 Duplex collecting system, US image.

• Clinical picture of urinary retention, distended bladder on US: proceed to urethral or suprapubic catheterization.

• Inadequate scan, other pathology (e.g. multiple cysts, duplex collecting system (Fig. 7.11), bladder wall thickening or mass) or other question (e.g. are there urinary flow jets visible in the bladder): arrange further imaging (e.g. CT or formal US).

Summary

➡ US scanning of the kidneys and bladder is rapid, safe and easy to learn.

➡ Inability to view the kidneys adequately should prompt the clinician to arrange formal US.

➡ Other disease entities (such as symptomatic AAA) must also be considered in patients with presumptive diagnosis of ureteric colic.

8

Gall bladder and common bile duct

Justin Bowra

Introduction

Gallstone disease is common and responsible for a range of emergency presentations. Ultrasound (US) scanning of the gall bladder (GB) and common bile duct (CBD) is relatively easy to learn, particularly for emergency physicians who are trained in focused assessment with sonography in trauma (FAST).

Why use US?

US is sensitive in the detection of the following:
- gallstones
- acute cholecystitis
- CBD dilatation.

Anatomy

The GB has a capacity of about 50 mL. It lies in the GB fossa below the liver, between the liver's right and quadrate lobes. It may be divided into neck, body and fundus.

GB size varies greatly, but most would agree it is distended if its transverse diameter >4 cm and if its total length is greater than that of the adjacent kidney. Distension strongly suggests an impacting gallstone.

The GB fundus projects below the liver (surface marking: intersection of costal margin and lateral border right rectus sheath). However, the exact position and shape of the fundus varies with its volume, patient anatomy and fasting status (Fig. 8.1). The GB body is the continuation of the fundus and narrows towards the neck, which continues into the cystic duct. The GB neck has the most constant position, related to the portal vein via the major lobar fissure.

In the biliary tree the cystic duct is 2–3 cm long (but variable) and has a normal diameter of 2 mm or less. It joins the common hepatic duct (formed by the union of the right and left hepatic ducts) to form the CBD. The CBD is normally 6 mm diameter or less. It descends in the hepatoduodenal ligament, anterior to the portal vein (PV) and to the right of the hepatic artery. It joins the pancreatic duct at the ampulla of Vater, which opens into the duodenum. On US, the CBD is best seen by tracing the major lobar fissure from

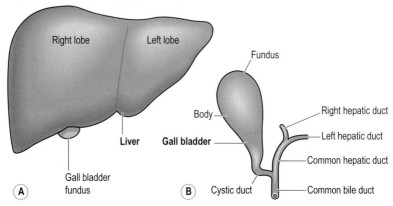

Fig. 8.1 Gall bladder anatomy. (A) Anterior aspect: gall bladder fundus projecting below liver. (B) Gall bladder and extrahepatic biliary tree.

the GB fossa to the PV, then looking just anterior to the PV.

What emergency US can tell you

- Is there a stone in the GB? Stones appear bright (echodense) with posterior acoustic shadowing.
- False negative for gallstones: small stones (<5 mm diameter) will not cast shadows.
- False positive for gallstones: air in the duodenum adjacent to GB may cast a 'dirty' shadow.
- Is the GB inflamed? Acute cholecystitis usually is caused by gallstone impaction of the GB neck or cystic duct. Diagnosis requires a combination of the following, as each individual finding may be found in other disease states:
  - Clinical features (e.g. fever and right upper quadrant pain and tenderness).

- Sonographic Murphy's sign (see below).
- Impacted gallstone: present except for rare cases, but may be difficult to view if in the cystic duct. Acalculous cholecystitis is rare but carries a worse prognosis.
- GB wall thickening >3 mm.
- Pericholecystic fluid.
- Is the CBD dilated? This is a crucial question in the patient with a picture of cholangitis or jaundice. Although it can be hard for US to demonstrate the obstructing stone, it is fairly easy to image the CBD as it runs in front of the portal vein.
- Is there a stone in the CBD? Usually a combination of luck and expertise is required to image CBD stones. Their presence may be inferred by a dilated CBD, but recall the many other causes of

dilated CBD (e.g. extrinsic compression from carcinoma).

What emergency US can't tell you

- Can I exclude a stone in the GB? Several views are required to completely exclude small GB calculi. However, small asymptomatic stones are of little clinical concern to the emergency department (ED) clinician.
- Can I exclude a CBD stone? The course of the CBD makes it very difficult to visualize its whole length, particularly the distal CBD.
- Other pathology such as intrahepatic biliary dilatation or liver parenchymal disease. Emergency US is not a substitute for a formal hepatobiliary US. For example, the liver has several segments which require experience to visualize adequately. The bile ducts are tubular structures and are found with blood vessels which they may resemble, so experience and Doppler are required to confidently identify the intrahepatic bile ducts.

 Formal upper abdominal US is complex and includes assessment of the liver parenchyma, intrahepatic bile ducts, pancreas and other structures. Stick to the gall bladder and common bile duct!

The technique and views

Patient position, probe and scanner settings

- As for FAST (Ch. 4, *FAST and EFAST*).
- Supine position is most practical in the unwell patient. However, if possible, a thorough examination will include imaging the patient in full inspiration and in the left lateral decubitus, as for cardiac scanning (Ch. 6, *Focused echocardiography and volume assessment*). In this position, a poorly visualized GB may drop into view.
- Alternative patient positions (such as right lateral and even erect) are sometimes required to completely view the GB.
- Fasting status: the GB contracts with meals and therefore is harder to view if the patient has recently eaten.

Probe placement and landmarks

1. Most ED sonologists prefer to commence with the probe aligned longitudinally in the mid-axillary line, at the costal margin or just subcostal (as for FAST). If doing so, identify the landmarks: right kidney, liver and diaphragm (highly echogenic) (Ch. 4, *FAST and EFAST*). Alter the probe angle to scan between the ribs, and scan through the phases of respiration to help you see the GB.

Fig. 8.2 Subcostal sweep.

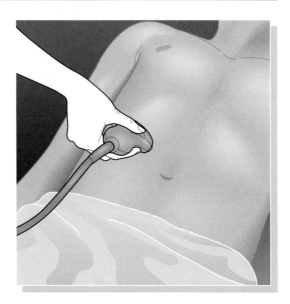

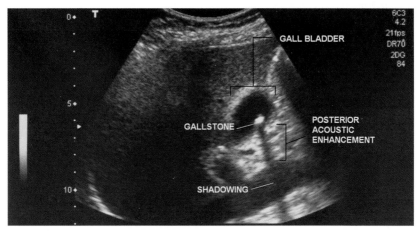

Fig. 8.3 Calculus in gall bladder with posterior acoustic enhancement from fluid, and posterior acoustic shadowing from stone, US image.

2. A more useful method is to place the probe medially in the subcostal position and 'sweep' down and laterally, just under the costal margin, angled upwards (Fig. 8.2). This technique and probe position are optimal for quick identification of the GB,

required for the radiological Murphy's sign, and best for CBD visualization, both described below.

3. The fasted GB appears as a well-demarcated fluid-filled structure inferior to the liver (Fig. 8.3). Alter depth and focus

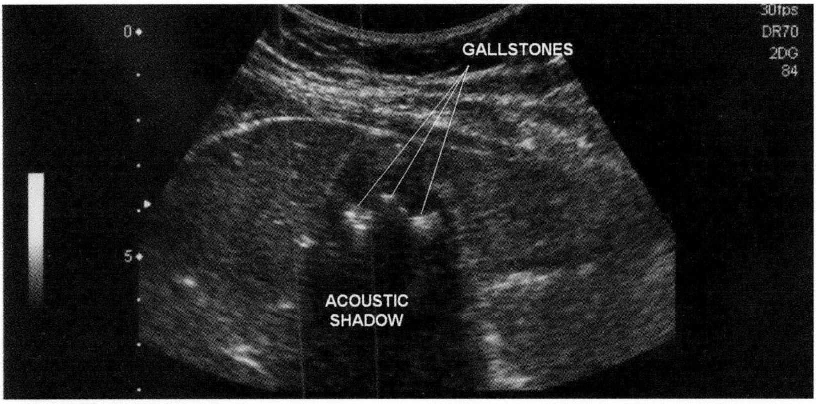

Fig. 8.4 Multiple gallstones, US image.

settings to maximize your view of the GB. Scan through the GB by altering probe angle and position and obtain longitudinal and transverse views of the GB. Be sure to scan as much of the GB as possible, to avoid missing localized pathology.

4. Is this the GB? Confirm the fluid-filled structure is indeed the GB (and not a loop of bowel) by scanning in two planes and by demonstrating the GB neck narrowing towards the cystic duct, or by the presence of calculi, or the absence of peristalsis.

5. GB calculi appear as highly reflective echoes with posterior acoustic shadows unless very small (<5 mm diameter) (Figs 8.3 and 8.4). They may roll into view when the patient moves into the left lateral position. Echoes which do not cast shadows usually represent sludge (Fig. 8.5).

6. To diagnose an impacted gallstone, scan the patient in more than one position (e.g. decubitus). An impacted gallstone does not move with gravity.

7. Sonographic Murphy's sign: with the probe in the subcostal position over the GB fundus, apply pressure. If this reproduces a patient's abdominal pain, this strongly suggests GB disease as the cause of the patient's symptoms.

8. GB wall:
   • Thickness: normal adult wall thickness is 3 mm or less. A thickened wall often appears as two echogenic lines with a hypoechoic region between them (Figs 8.6 and 8.7). This suggests acute inflammation and oedema but may also be found in other disease states (e.g. congestive cardiac failure and sepsis). In addition, normal non-fasted

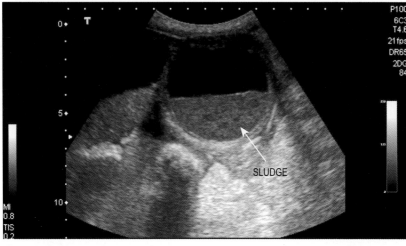

Fig. 8.5 Gall bladder sludge, US image, courtesy of Dr Rob Reardon.

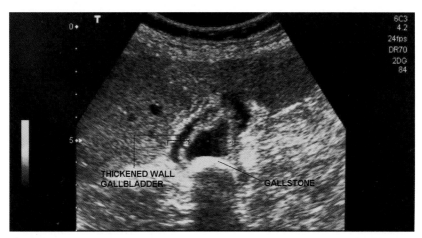

Fig. 8.6 Acute cholecystitis and impacted stone, transverse view, US image. Gall bladder wall thickening with localized free fluid.

GB walls will also be thickened due to contraction. This is important to remember in the non-fasted ED population.

- Other wall findings, such as focal wall thickening (e.g. carcinoma) or calcification can be found in a variety of diseases which are beyond the scope of this book. GB polyps are a not infrequent finding, and can be distinguished from calculi by the fact that they are usually small, solitary or small in number, are non-mobile

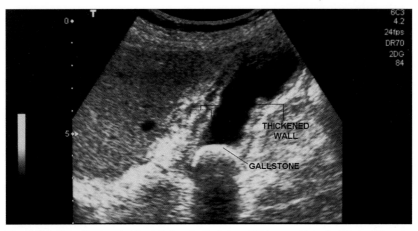

Fig. 8.7 Same patient as in Fig. 8.6, longitudinal view, US image. Note that the gallstone's posterior shadowing in both images is less obvious because of concomitant acoustic enhancement due to fluid and liver. Solution: decrease gain.

and attached to the wall, and do not shadow.

9. Air in the GB lumen or wall: emphysematous cholecystitis is a rare surgical emergency. Air in the lumen is usually hyperechoic but without posterior shadowing. Air in the walls may simulate calcification.

10. Free fluid (FF) around the GB: localized fluid around the GB is usually found in acute cholecystitis (particularly with GB perforation) but may be found in other disease states such as pancreatitis.

11. CBD: at the porta hepatis, this runs along and anterior to the portal vein, therefore this is usually the best place to measure it.

   • Identify the portal vein first: with the probe in the subcostal position, change probe angle to align it along an imaginary line between the axilla and umbilicus (Fig. 8.8).

   • Ask the patient to hold his/her breath in full inspiration. This brings the structures into better view and allows the use of Doppler without movement artefact.

   • Identify the GB neck then the portal triad. The large portal vein with its echogenic walls is usually easy to identify, anterior to the inferior vena cava (IVC). The CBD lies along the front of the vein, is smaller calibre and has very echogenic walls. The right hepatic artery crosses between the two, so use colour and/or spectral Doppler to distinguish the vessels (Fig. 8.9).

   • Measure the internal diameter of the CBD where its internal

Fig. 8.8 Probe position for common bile duct.

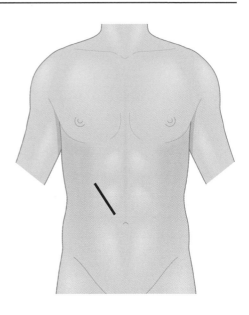

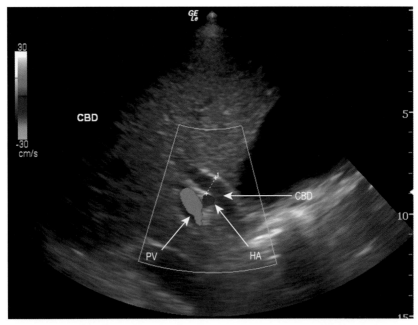

Fig. 8.9 Portal vein (PV), hepatic artery (HA) and common bile duct (CBD), US image. Doppler scan confirms flow in PV and HA.

diameter is greatest and ideally just at or above the point where the hepatic artery crosses between CBD and portal vein. If CBD diameter is greater than 6 mm this suggests CBD dilatation. Other causes include increasing age and post-cholecystectomy state.

Handy hints and caveats

✓ The GB is most easily seen in the fasted patient. Beware physiological GB wall thickening in the non-fasted patient.

✓ If the patient can lie in left lateral position and hold his/her breath in full inspiration, this will improve your view.

✓ Congenital variations (such as duplication) are rare.

✓ More than one window, scanning plane and patient position are required to view the GB adequately.

✓ In itself, the presence of stones does not infer cholecystitis. Asymptomatic stones are a common incidental finding.

✓ Similarly, GB wall thickening alone may be found in other disease states besides acute cholecystitis:

✓ non-fasting state

✓ ascites

✓ systemic oedema (e.g. congestive cardiac failure)

✓ cancer (if localized).

✓ To find a really small gallstone in GB:

✓ turn down the power (too strong an US beam makes small shadows 'disappear')

✓ turn up the frequency

✓ turn off the compounding.

✓ An impacted stone in the cystic duct may be difficult for the ED sonographer to detect. Therefore, if the other clinical and sonographic features of acute cholecystitis are present, the diagnosis may be inferred.

✓ Occasionally, a GB becomes completely filled with gallstones. When this occurs, the normal fluid-filled structure with posterior enhancement is no longer seen. Instead, two parallel bright lines with posterior shadowing are seen. This represents wall-echo shadow (WES). The bright line nearer the probe is the GB wall. The line beneath represents the echogenic stone. In multiple stones this second line is often irregular (Fig. 8.10).

✓ WES is important because it may be misinterpreted as a bowel loop but in fact represents cholelithiasis.

✓ Inability to view the GB, or abnormal findings such as focal wall thickening or calcification, should prompt the clinician to arrange formal radiological investigation such as US or CT.

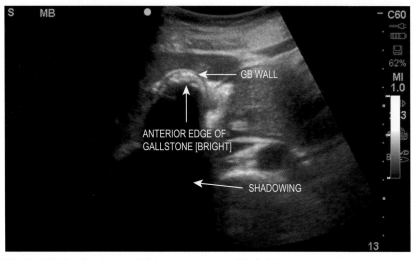

Fig. 8.10 Wall-echo shadow, US image, courtesy of Dr Rob Reardon.

 Diagnosis of acute cholecystitis requires a *combination* of clinical signs (e.g. sonographic Murphy's sign) and US findings (e.g. calculi, GB wall thickening and pericholecystic fluid).

 Gallstones are a common incidental finding. In isolation, their presence does not infer cholecystitis or biliary colic.

Now what?

- Acute cholecystitis, or features of cholangitis with dilated CBD: commence intravenous antibiotics and consult a surgeon immediately.

- Clinical picture of biliary colic, gallstones demonstrated: discuss with a surgeon.

- No features of GB disease, sonographic Murphy's negative: seek other cause of patient's symptoms.

- Inadequate scan, more complex pathology sought or clinical picture of biliary disease and unable to detect gallstones: arrange formal US.

Summary

➡ US scanning of the GB is rapid and easy to learn.

➡ CBD is harder to scan and requires practice and good technique.

➡ US is sensitive in the detection of GB calculi, acute cholecystitis and dilated CBD.

➡ Emergency US is not a substitute for formal sonography.

➡ Inability to view the GB, or abnormal findings such as focal wall thickening or calcification should prompt the clinician to arrange formal US.

9 Early pregnancy

Sabrina Kuah, Justin Bowra, Tony Joseph

Introduction

The symptoms of an ectopic pregnancy (EP) (e.g. abdominal pain, amenorrhoea and vaginal bleeding in a patient with a positive pregnancy test) can be difficult to distinguish from other complications of early pregnancy such as spontaneous abortion, ruptured corpus luteum cyst or unrelated illness such as acute appendicitis. Likewise, examination may prove unremarkable, especially with an early unruptured EP. Ultrasound (US) is non-invasive and can be performed with little delay (during resuscitation of the patient if necessary) and correlated with a quantitative serum beta human chorionic gonadotrophin (βHCG). Serial US and βHCG are essential for monitoring equivocal cases.

Ectopic pregnancy

An ectopic pregnancy (EP) can be defined as implantation of a pregnancy outside the uterine cavity. Its incidence varies geographically from 1 in 28 to 1 in 300 pregnancies (19 per 1000 pregnancies in USA), with 65% occurring in the 25–34 age group. Ninety-eight per cent occur in the fallopian tube with the remainder being abdominal, ovarian, cervical or even in the caesarean section scar.

Despite early detection due to transvaginal US (TVS) and βHCG, EP remains the leading cause of pregnancy-related maternal death in the first trimester, accounting for about 10% of all pregnancy-related deaths.

Risk factors for EP include previous EP (odds ratio (OR) 8.3), tubal pathology (OR 3.5–25) and previous tubal surgery (OR 21).

Two to three per cent of EP may be interstitial. In these cases, the EP is located in the interstitial part of the fallopian tube as it transverses the uterine wall, and the main part of the gestational sac is located outside the uterine cavity. The mortality of these pregnancies is twice that of other tubal pregnancies (2%) as they tend to rupture later (at 8–16 weeks gestation).

Heterotopic pregnancy (defined as co-existing intrauterine and extrauterine pregnancy) is rare: 1 in 30 000 spontaneous conceptions and 1 : 100

to 1 : 3000 technically assisted conceptions.

Why use US?

Bedside US is safe and can be performed at the bedside without interrupting patient resuscitation. Two methods are used: transabdominal (TA) and transvaginal (TV). The TV method is more accurate and achieves better resolution of pelvic structures (Figs 9.1–9.3). Unlike TA scanning, it does not require a full bladder. However, TV scanning is invasive, requires verbal patient consent and needs more exhaustive training than TA and consequently is outside the scope of this text.

One advantage of TA over TV scanning is its ability to assess the abdomen and upper pelvis. Pathology here may be missed on a TV scan, because the higher-frequency transducer limits the depth of view to the lower pelvis.

A TA scan performed by an emergency physician does not seek to replace a formal US study. It is an on-the-spot tool to assist in the assessment of early pregnancy. For example, it may be used to identify patients with a definite *in utero* pregnancy (IUP). Given the rare incidence of heterotopic pregnancy, a stable uncomplicated patient with a live IUP demonstrated on US is a good candidate for discharge with appropriate follow-up.

Conversely, all patients with an equivocal US (i.e. one in which a definite IUP is not identified) require a gynaecological (OG) consultation.

Studies indicate that US-trained emergency department (ED) physicians can reliably determine the

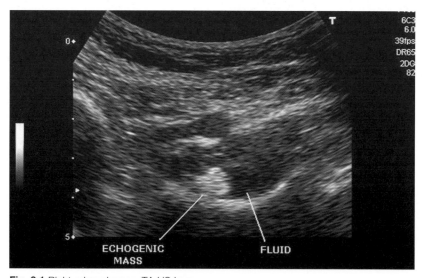

Fig. 9.1 Right adnexal mass, TA US image.

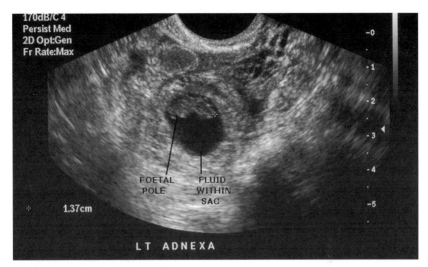

Fig. 9.2 Ectopic pregnancy, TV US image.

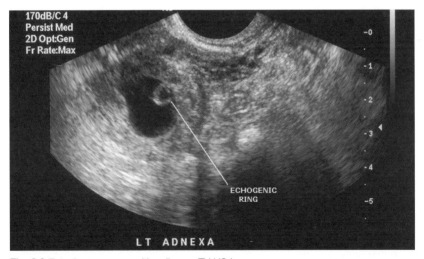

Fig. 9.3 Ectopic pregnancy with yolk sac, TV US image.

presence of an IUP. It has been observed that screening ultrasounds performed in this context can decrease ED stay by almost 120 minutes. A significant decrease in missed EP has been observed when US-trained ED physicians performed a screening US prior to selecting patients appropriate for discharge from the ED.

What emergency US can tell you

- Is there an EP? Most EPs will *not* demonstrate an extrauterine gestational sac containing a yolk sac or embryo. However, the finding of an adnexal mass in a patient with an empty uterus and elevated βHCG makes EP likely.
- Is there free fluid (FF)? US can detect the presence of FF in the pouch of Douglas, which may be due to a bleeding EP or a haemorrhagic/ruptured cyst. In the supine patient, FF also collects in Morison's pouch and/or the lienorenal interface, so many ED sonologists will include a focused assessment with sonography in trauma FAST scan in their assessment (see Ch. 4, *FAST and EFAST*).
- Is the uterus empty? An empty uterus in a woman with a positive pregnancy test is highly suggestive of an EP.
- Is there an IUP? Except in the rare incidence of heterotopic pregnancy (beware assisted reproduction treatment patients), identification of an IUP excludes EP.
- Is there a foetal heartbeat (FHB)? It is fairly easy to detect FHB as a 'flicker' on two-dimensional (2D) images.
- What is the foetal heart rate (FHR)? This can be assessed using M-mode (see below).

What emergency US can't tell you

- Is the IUP normal? Leave comments such as 'normal pregnancy' to the formal sonographers. However, the presence of a true gestational sac, foetal pole and FHB are reassuring features (Table 9.1).
- What is the gestational age? Although it is possible to estimate this using measures such as crown–rump length, most ED sonologists (including the authors) recommend that this is left to the experts.
- If I demonstrate an IUP, can I rule out an EP completely? Not always. For example, an *interstitial* pregnancy can be difficult to distinguish from an IUP that is eccentrically placed—look for a gestational sac or hyperechoic mass in the cornua with myometrial thinning. A hyperechoic 'interstitial line' may be seen extending from the uterine cavity to the cornual gestational sac. If in doubt, arrange formal US.

The role of βHCG

Of all the laboratory parameters which may discriminate between a viable IUP and an EP, βHCG is the most useful. In the presence of a pregnancy, βHCG can be detected prior to a missed menses and can remain elevated for weeks after pregnancy demise.

Table 9.1 Transabdominal (TA) findings in normal pregnancy

Approx. 5 weeks, βHCG >1800 IU	Gestational sac (including yolk sac). Yolk sac should be seen by 7 weeks in normal IUP.
7 weeks	Foetal pole (should be visible when mean gestational sac measurement is >25 mm). Embryo should be seen by 8 weeks.
7 weeks	Foetal cardiac activity (note: if you can see foetal pole on TA scan, you should always be able to detect cardiac activity).

Note that the timings indicated are estimates only and vary with patient habitus, machine quality and operator skill. All findings will appear earlier with TV scanning.
Note also that gestational age calculations based on last menstrual period (LMP) can be wrong!

When assessing serum βHCG, it is important to consider:

- The absolute level: Most viable IUP will be visible on TVS at a βHCG level of >1500 IU/L and TA scan at a βHCG >1800. Hence, if TA scan demonstrates an empty uterus and βHCG >1800, suspect EP. However, a level below 1500 must not be interpreted as 'no EP' or 'no risk of EP rupture'.

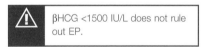

βHCG <1500 IU/L does not rule out EP.

- Whether the βHCG is rising or falling: for example, in the case above (βHCG >1500, empty uterus), if this is a wanted pregnancy in a stable patient, the OG team may elect to repeat the βHCG and TVS in 2 days. A falling βHCG is consistent with a failed pregnancy (non-viable IUP, tubal abortion, spontaneously resolving EP).

- The *rate of decline:* βHCG falls *more slowly* with an EP than with a completed abortion. Hence, if the βHCG falls by more than 50% in 48 hours in the presence of an indeterminate US, an EP is very unlikely, and most likely there is a spontaneous abortion.

- The *rate of rise:* 85% of viable IUP demonstrate a mean doubling time of 1.4 to 2.1 days until day 40 when βHCG reaches a plateau of 100 000. While this can also be said for a minority of EP, the rise in βHCG in most patients with EP is much slower. Hence, if the βHCG is *failing to double* over 72 hours and repeat TVS shows an empty uterus, the pregnancy is non-viable regardless of location and treatment for EP can be initiated as appropriate.

Conversely, a normal rise in βHCG needs to be monitored with serial TVS until the location of the gestation can be visualized.

Clinical picture

- The patient: female and fertile.
- Pregnancy: always assume a woman of child-bearing age is pregnant and test serum βHCG.

- Classic features such as pain, shock and vaginal bleeding may not be present.

 If in doubt, assume the patient has EP until proven otherwise.

Before you scan

- Initial resuscitation as clinically indicated.
- Get help: the doctor performing the scan should not also be resuscitating the patient.
- If the patient is unstable, contact OG before you scan.
- Send blood for full blood count, quantitative βHCG and either group and hold or crossmatch as indicated.

The technique and views: TA scan

Patient position

- Supine is most practical.
- Full bladder if possible. (It is possible to perform TA scan without a full bladder if you do not have time to allow the bladder to fill, but the results will be much harder to interpret.) Consider referral for TV scan or urgent OG review in such situations.
- A bimanual pelvic examination prior to an US examination is useful; for example, localization of a mass or tenderness may direct a TA scan.

Probe and scanner settings

- Most portable US machines have obstetric preset. If unavailable, use standard abdominal preset.
- Curved probe: suggested frequency 2.5–5 MHz.
- Begin with standard B-mode setting.
- M-mode also should be used to demonstrate the FHB.
- Standard orientation: patient's right is on *left* of screen.
- Adjust image depth and focus according to patient habitus.

Probe placement and landmarks

- Commence with the probe in the midline just above the pubis (see Figs 4.11 and 4.14). Identify the bladder (as in Ch. 4). Use the full bladder as a sonographic 'window' to deeper structures.
- Scanning transversely and longitudinally, identify the uterus as it lies behind the bladder, documenting its size, shape and orientation (Fig. 9.4). Alter image depth and focus as required. In pregnancy, the uterus appears as a thick-walled, hollow muscular structure with non-echogenic fluid. The normal non-pregnant uterus in a woman of child-bearing age is less than 10 cm long and less than 6 cm in width. Identify the myometrium, endometrium (which appears as a thin, hyperechoic line) and cervix.
- Focus on the uterine cavity: scan longitudinally and transversely

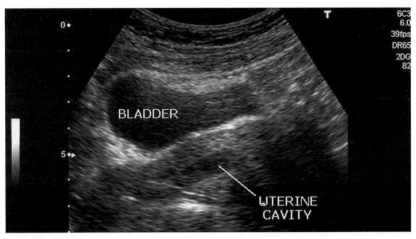

Fig. 9.4 Empty uterus longitudinal section, TA scan, US image. Gestational age 6 weeks, positive pregnancy test. TV scan demonstrated ectopic pregnancy.

through the cavity for evidence of an IUP: an intrauterine gestational sac with a yolk sac, foetal pole or cardiac motion.

- Use M-mode to measure FHR. (See below for details.)
- Then identify the two ovaries, which appear oval and hypoechoic. Ideally, one should document their volume in millilitres (mL). However, the details of ovarian volume measurement are beyond the scope of this text.
- Unlike the ovaries, fallopian tubes are not usually visible unless dilated.
- The adnexae are not seen as a specific structure on TA US.
- Evaluate the cul-de-sac for free fluid (FF), echogenic rings and masses.
- Use gentle probe pressure and angling to differentiate any pathological structure (such as a

ring or mass) from ovarian pathology such as a ruptured corpus luteum. Identify whether any pathological structure moves independently of the ovary. (Often this is easier to demonstrate transvaginally.)

- Finally, methodically sweep through the lower abdomen and pelvis. Pathology here may be missed by TV scans, which concentrate on the lower pelvis.
- A modified FAST (see Ch. 4) may identify FF elsewhere in the abdomen. Free intraperitoneal fluid in a patient receiving ART and complaining of abdominal pain may represent ovarian hyperstimulation, but a ruptured EP must be assumed first.

Essential views and findings

- Normal IUP: this usually excludes EP (except in the rare circumstance

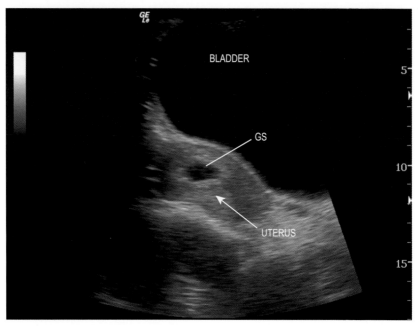

Fig. 9.5 Gestational sac (GS), TA US image.

of heterotopic pregnancy). A normal IUP should demonstrate the following:

- *True gestational sac* (Fig. 9.5): this is the first true sign of pregnancy on US and represents the chorionic cavity (sac itself), implanting chorionic villi and associated decidual tissue (outer echogenic region). Initially it appears as an echogenic ring, representing a small fluid-filled sac embedded below the midline. As it enlarges, it becomes more elliptical. Initially there is nothing distinctively visible in the sac cavity. Hence, it may be confused with a pseudosac (see below).

- The spherical *yolk sac* should be taken as the first *definite* sign of pregnancy on US. It is the first anatomic structure seen inside a gestational sac and may be seen from a mean sac diameter (MSD) of 5 mm, although it may not appear until MSD 8 mm. When first visible on US it is a perfect echogenic ring inside the gestational sac. This combination of a hyperechoic 'ring' (the yolk sac) within the hyperechoic outer gestational sac is known as the 'double decidual sac' sign (Fig. 9.6).

- By contrast, the *pseudosac* (pseudogestational sac) has only a single hyperechoic layer, no

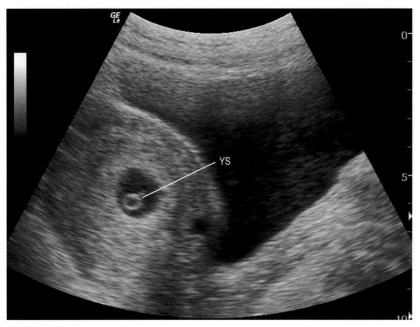

Fig. 9.6 Yolk sac (YS), US image.

yolk sac 'ring' within it, no foetal pole and no cardiac activity. It is seen in 10–20% of EP due to the hormonal changes in pregnancy and may display a low-level echo pattern due to debris in its cavity, particularly in patients with a high βHCG level (Fig. 9.7).

- At 6 weeks the embryonic disc (thickened region at the edge of the yolk sac) may be visible with the foetal pole and cardiac activity (M-mode) detectable from 7 weeks (Fig. 9.8).
- Eventually the foetus begins to have a recognizable appearance (Fig. 9.9).
- The yolk sac continues to grow to a maximum diameter of 6 mm by 10 weeks, all the while migrating to the periphery until it is no longer visible by the end of the first trimester.
- FHB: This may be visible as a rapid 'flicker' within the foetal pole. If M-mode is available, direct the scanning line through the foetal pole to demonstrate cardiac activity and measure FHR (Fig. 9.10). Most portable US machines have the software to calculate FHR. Follow the instructions in the user manual for details.
- *Do not use Doppler* when scanning in pregnancy, as there may be a risk of danger to the foetus.
- US findings in EP:
  1. An embryo with cardiac activity outside the uterus is diagnostic

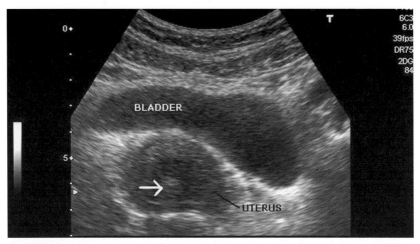

Fig. 9.7 Pseudosac, US image.

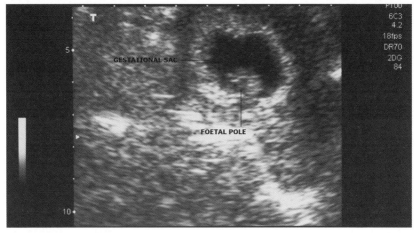

Fig. 9.8 Foetal pole/heartbeat, US image.

but only found in 8–26% of EP (Fig. 9.2).

2. More commonly (40–70%) an 'echogenic ring' is visualized outside the uterus (Fig. 9.3).

3. The combination of an echogenic adnexal mass, an empty uterus and a positive pregnancy test carries 85% likelihood of EP.

4. A ruptured EP may appear as a complex adnexal mass of mixed echogenicity.

5. An *empty uterus* alone (or pseudogestational sac) is suggestive of EP but may represent other states such as

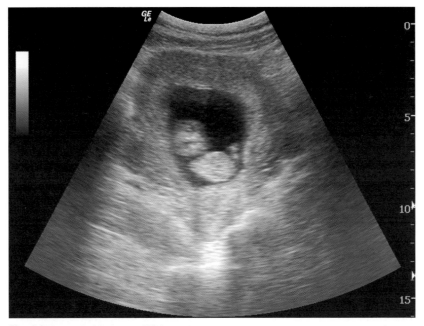

Fig. 9.9 Recognizable foetus, US image.

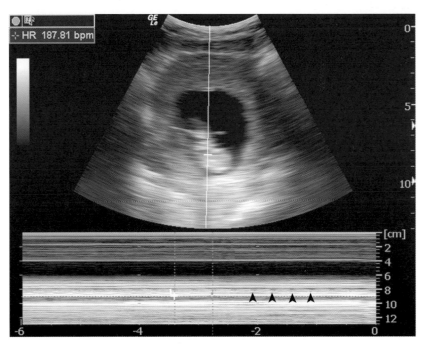

Fig. 9.10 Foetal heart rate measured, M-mode US image. Heartbeat is seen as regular 'wave' (arrowheads).

miscarriage or even early normal IUP (Fig. 9.4).

6. Intraperitoneal haemorrhage can result in cul-de-sac fluid, which may be particulate depending on its age. The combination of positive pregnancy test, FF and an empty uterus carries a 71% risk of EP. This rises to 95% if a large amount of FF is present.

7. The combination of an echogenic mass and FF makes EP almost certain.

8. An ovarian EP can be difficult to distinguish from a haemorrhagic corpus luteum or corpus luteum cyst as both will move with the ovary. If available, colour Doppler demonstrates a 'ring of fire' around the highly vascular, usually viable trophoblastic tissue of an EP. However, to a lesser extent, a corpus luteum may have a similar appearance.

9. Interstitial EPs are richly vascular and can remain viable for some time, growing to a large size. Initially appearing as an asymmetrical IUP, the cornual ectopic is not actually within the uterine cavity. Look for a hyperechoic 'interstitial line' extending from the uterine cavity to the cornual gestational sac.

10. Likewise a cervical EP is not in the uterine cavity (differential diagnosis: imminent miscarriage).

11. Twenty to thirty per cent of EP have no detectable sonographic abnormalities at the time of diagnosis.

Handy hints

✓ If in doubt, assume the patient has EP until proven otherwise.

✓ Urgently refer all shocked patients with suspected EP to the gynaecologists. Do not waste time performing a TA scan before referral.

✓ You are not a sonographer! Refer all indeterminate scans for formal US or urgent OG review, as dictated by clinical picture.

✓ A full bladder is required for best results in a TA scan. If empty, either push fluids or refer for TV scan.

✓ Hence, if EP is suspected as a possibility, it is reasonable to perform an US regardless of βHCG level.

✓ Due to inter-assay variability (10–15% variability), serial monitoring should take place in the same laboratory.

✓ When measuring FHR, use M-mode *not pulsed Doppler*. Pulsed Doppler may adversely affect the foetus.

✓ *False positives for EP*

  ✓ Early normal IUP (prior to appearance of yolk sac)

  ✓ Miscarriage

  ✓ Corpus luteum cyst.

✓ *False negatives for EP*
  ✓ Intrauterine pseudosac
  ✓ Interstitial EP
  ✓ Heterotopic pregnancy (extremely rare). Such patients usually have had assisted reproduction.

 If in doubt, assume the patient has EP until proven otherwise.

Now what?

- Unstable patient: resuscitate and notify OG immediately.
  - If EP is suspected or identified, the patient must be transferred immediately to operating theatre (OT).
  - If unable to rule out EP, decision to proceed to OT (or further imaging) must be based on clinical likelihood of EP.
- Stable patient, IUP confirmed, no risk factors for heterotopia: EP effectively has been ruled out. Refer for outpatient OG review.

- Stable patient, IUP confirmed, but patient has risk factors for heterotopia: further assessment as for EP.
- Stable patient, βHCG >1800, empty uterus and/or other suspicious findings such as adnexal mass on TA scan: suspect EP and notify OG.
- Stable patient, βHCG <1800, empty uterus: this is a complex situation and must be discussed with OG. TV scan should be performed by OG or radiology department. If TV scan is also negative, local practices will differ. Options include monitoring the patient and repeating βHCG and TVS in 2–3 days.

 Beware the pseudosac!

Summary

TA scanning by ED physicians is not a substitute for formal US. However, in conjunction with serum βHCG, it is an invaluable tool in the ED to assist diagnosis of abdominal pain or vaginal bleeding in the first trimester.

10 Ultrasound-guided procedures

Justin Bowra

This chapter covers the following procedures:

- probe sterilization
- vascular access
- thoracocentesis
- pericardiocentesis
- paracentesis
- suprapubic catheterization
- lumbar puncture.

Nerve blocks are covered separately in Chapter 11.

Why use ultrasound?

Even with an expert knowledge of anatomy, blind insertion of needles and drainage catheters can be dangerous and technically difficult for many reasons such as abnormal anatomy and coagulopathy.

Where available and practical, ultrasound (US)-guided needle insertion is best practice. It enables accurate location of the relevant anatomy, identifies local pathology such as thrombosed veins and decreases the risk of complications such as damage to nearby structures.

Several studies have demonstrated that central venous cannulation

(CVC) using two-dimensional (2D) US guidance is safer and more successful than the landmark technique.

In the UK, current National Institute for Health and Clinical Excellence (NICE) guidelines (www.nice.org.uk) recommend 2D US guidance for emergency and elective CVC.

Probe sterilization

- Sterilize the probe with the aid of an assistant. One method is to prepare the probe with standard gel, then insert the probe into a sterile US probe sheath or a sterile glove and apply sterile gel over the sheath (Fig. 10.1).
- An alternative method is the 'gel-free technique':
  - Cover the probe with standard gel as above, then with a sterile adherent dressing such as Opsite 3000® (Fig. 10.2). Ensure that no air bubbles are trapped between the probe and the dressing, or the resulting US image will be affected.

Fig. 10.1 Covering probe with sterile dressing.

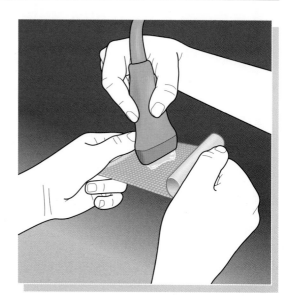

Fig. 10.2 Second dressing wrapped around probe.

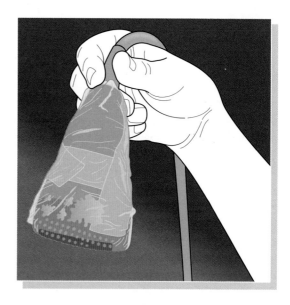

- Instead of using sterile gel over this, as a scanning medium simply use the antiseptic liquid used to sterilize your field (e.g. chlorhexidine).

- The resulting image will be adequate for most procedures, and the technique is less messy (Figs 10.3 and 10.4).

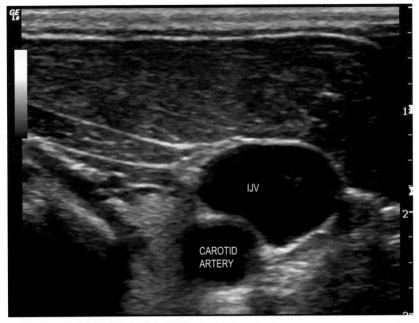

Fig. 10.3 Right internal jugular vein (IJV) using sterile gel, US image.

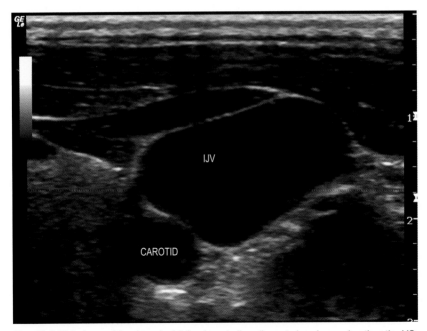

Fig. 10.4 Right internal jugular vein (IJV) using sterile adherent dressing and antiseptic, US image.

When preparing a sterile probe, it is easy to accidentally contaminate your gloves, so wear a double set.

Central venous cannulation

Anatomy

The internal jugular vein (IJV) runs in the carotid sheath, usually lateral to the common carotid artery (CCA) and deep to the sternocleidomastoid muscle (SCM) (Fig. 10.5). Its compressibility and relative safety make it a preferred CVC site in the emergency department (ED). A traditional cannulation site is approximately halfway between the sternal notch and the mastoid process, at the bifurcation of the SCM.

As well as compressibility, the femoral vein (FV; also known as common femoral vein) has the advantage of distance from important structures such as the airway and lungs. In the femoral sheath it is usually medial to the pulsation of the femoral artery, which lies approximately halfway between the symphysis pubis and the anterior superior iliac spine (ASIS) (Fig. 10.6).

Subclavian vein cannulation is technically difficult and beyond the scope of this text.

It is essential to distinguish between veins and arteries on US:

- Vein larger, oval cross-section, thinner walled and compressible (unless thrombus or proximal obstruction, e.g. massive pulmonary embolus, PE).
- Diameter of vein changes with respiration and Valsalva.
- Arterial pulsation (beware transmitted venous pulsation).

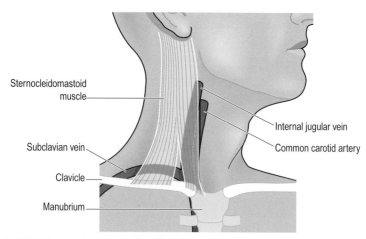

Sternocleidomastoid muscle

Subclavian vein

Clavicle

Manubrium

Internal jugular vein

Common carotid artery

Fig. 10.5 Relations of right internal jugular vein.

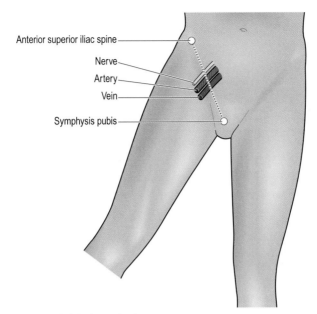

Anterior superior iliac spine
Nerve
Artery
Vein
Symphysis pubis

Fig. 10.6 Relations of right femoral vein.

- Doppler waveform analysis will further differentiate vein from artery. However, Doppler is not essential and not recommended by NICE.

Which technique?

Three techniques are described. A combination of all three is used by the author.

'Static' technique

US is used to identify the target vein and mark the optimum site of needle entry prior to sterile preparation of the field (Fig. 10.7). This confirms venous depth, course and compressibility. It is recommended as a 'screening exam' prior to using one of the other techniques below. Used alone, it is less technically demanding and obviates any requirement for sterility. However, it is not as safe as real-time US guidance.

Real-time in-plane and out-of-plane techniques

Described below, both techniques require a sterile technique. Both are more difficult than the static technique and an assistant is required to 'drive' the US machine. However, real-time US guidance is safer than the static approach.

 US may be used to mark the site for subsequent cannulation, then the probe is removed. However, real-time US guidance is safer.

Fig. 10.7 Initial probe placement for IJV.

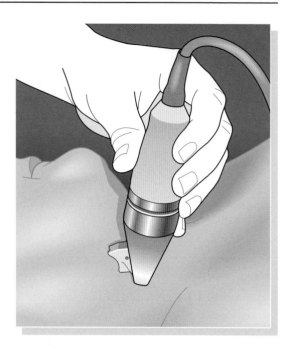

 In addition, all the usual risks, contraindications and complications of Seldinger CVC insertion apply.

CVC using real-time US

Preparation

- Informed consent unless emergency.

- Patient attached to monitors and oxygen. Local anaesthetic and Seldinger technique equipment.

- Situate US monitor in your line of sight: it is difficult and potentially hazardous to insert the cannula when craning to look over your shoulder at the screen.

- Choose site and confirm anatomy with static US, then prep and drape site.

Patient's position

- Dictated by clinical picture.

- IJV cannulation: 10 degrees Trendelenburg tilt will significantly increase IJV diameter and prevent intracranial air embolism.

- Femoral cannulation: leg abducted. Hang the leg over the edge of the bed if necessary.

Probe and scanner settings

- High-frequency (e.g. 7.5 MHz) linear array probe. Some probes have a notch in their midline to guide the needle.

- Vascular preset.

'Out-of-plane' or transverse technique

1. With your non-dominant hand, place probe transversely over the

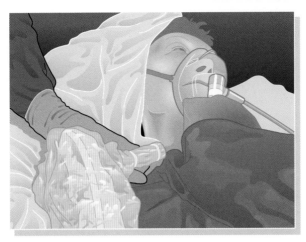

Fig. 10.8 Sterile probe placement, out-of-plane technique.

chosen site. Identify vein, artery and nearby structures on screen (Figs 10.3, 10.4 and 10.8). Lymph nodes may mimic vessels in cross-section but are not compressible or tubular. Use colour Doppler if in doubt.

2. Move probe and alter image depth and focus so that vein appears in the centre of the screen. This will serve as a landmark for needle position.

3. Administer local anaesthetic (LA) over the course of the vein at the probe's midway point. When LA has taken effect, a scalpel may be used to nick the skin to ease the subsequent passage of the introducer needle. This step is not essential.

4. With your dominant hand, insert introducer needle (attached to syringe) at the site of LA, at a steeper angle to the skin than that used for blind cannula insertion. Introduce the needle at an angle and position to ensure the needle tip intersects the vein in the plane of the US image and does not overshoot the plane of the US image (Figs 10.9 and 10.10). Using out-of-plane technique, the image of the needle often is not seen, but its ring-down artefact will confirm its position (Fig. 10.11). If in doubt, change the angle of the probe until the needle is seen (Fig. 10.12).

5. The major risk of such a steep angle is inadvertent 'through and through' venous puncture. Avoid this by the following:

• Introduce the needle more slowly than when performing blind cannula insertion.

• Introduce the needle under real-time visualization of the US image.

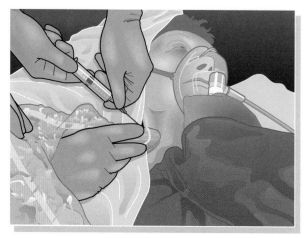

Fig. 10.9 Needle insertion, out-of-plane technique.

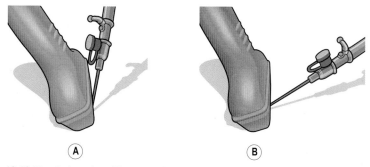

(A)   (B)

Fig. 10.10 Needle insertion: (A) correct, (B) incorrect.

- Watch for 'tenting' of the vein's upper wall inwards as the needle approaches the vein (Fig. 10.13). When the needle enters the vein, this tenting will diminish even if you do not see the needle in the vein. The needle tip (or its artefact) should be visible in the venous lumen (Fig. 10.14) but may not be if the US plane does not intersect the needle.

- Confirm position by aspirating venous blood.

- Once the needle has entered the vein, decrease the angle of the needle. Take care to ensure the needle tip remains in the lumen.

6. Remove the syringe and introduce the guidewire. The guidewire should be visible in the venous lumen. Using transverse and longitudinal scanning, trace the path of the guidewire to ensure it has not kinked back.

7. Remove the probe, complete Seldinger insertion of the cannula

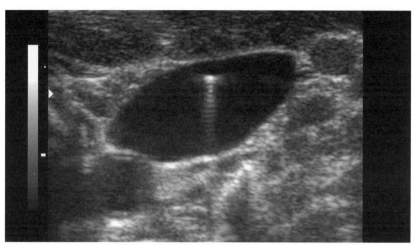

Fig. 10.11 Ring down using out-of-plane technique, US image.

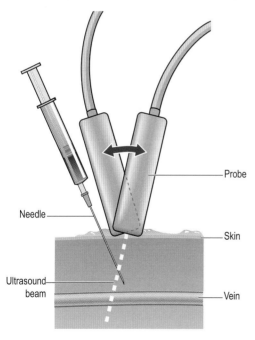

Fig. 10.12 Changing the angle of the probe until needle is visualized.

Needle

Probe

Skin

Ultrasound beam

Vein

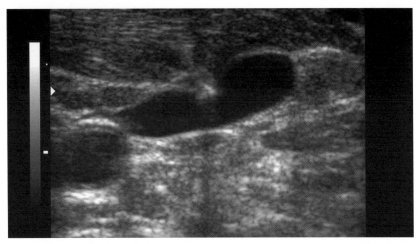

Fig. 10.13 'Tenting', US image.

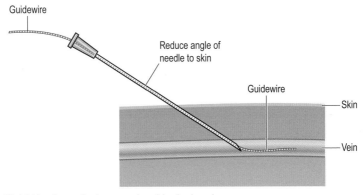

Fig. 10.14 Needle angle decreased, guidewire in vein.

and check position with X-ray as per local protocol.

'In-plane' or longitudinal section technique:

1. The same as for out-of-plane.
2. Once vein is identified, rotate the probe until the vein appears in longitudinal section (LS):

confirm the vessel is venous using the checklist above ('Anatomy') (Fig. 10.15).

3. Administer LA beneath the probe and consider nicking the skin with a scalpel as above.
4. Introduce introducer needle at a shallow angle as for traditional blind cannulation. This allows

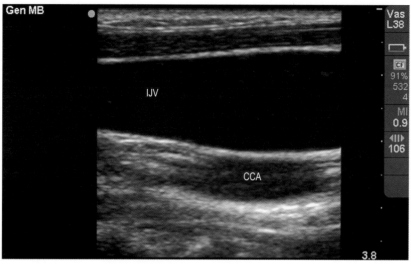

Fig. 10.15 Right IJV and CCA longitudinal view, US image.

easier visualization of the needle on US (Figs 10.16 and 10.17).

5. The major pitfall of this technique is inadvertently moving the probe so that its plane no longer parallels that of the vein and needle. This may lead to needle overshoot or even arterial cannulation.

6. Once the needle has entered the vein, complete steps 6 and 7 as above.

➡ Difficult to visualize US image of needle: 'ring down' artefact used instead.
➡ Risk of overshoot if probe plane does not intersect needle.

In-plane technique

➡ Shallow angle needle entry.
➡ Requires finer control of the probe to ensure that entire needle (especially tip) is on screen, but safer than out-of-plane technique.
➡ Risks if probe's plane no longer parallels that of the vein or needle: needle overshoot, arterial cannulation.
    A combination of a non-sterile screening exam, then a real-time technique, is safest.

Summary

Out-of-plane technique

➡ Steep angle needle entry.
➡ Easier and preferred by novice operators.

Handy hints and pitfalls

✓ Doppler is not required to distinguish veins from arteries.
✓ Keep the US screen directly in front, in your line of sight.

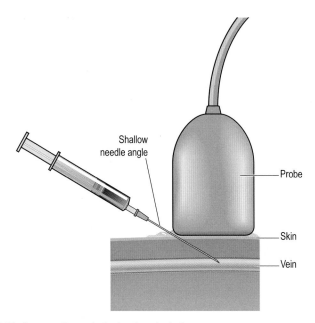

Fig. 10.16 Shallow needle angle for in-plane technique.

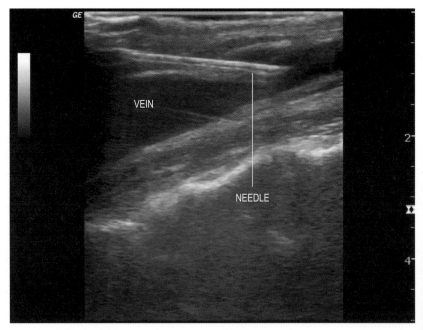

Fig. 10.17 Needle in IJV, in-plane technique, US image.

✓ You will need an assistant to drive the machine.

✓ Needle angle differs between in-plane and out-of-plane techniques.

✓ In-plane technique is safer but can be harder to learn.

✓ Avoid through-and-through venous puncture by:

✓ Slow needle insertion.

✓ Real-time US visualization.

✓ Keep the needle tip on screen (if using in-plane approach).

✓ Watch for tenting of vein as needle approaches.

✓ Continuous aspiration of syringe.

✓ US guidance may also be used when cannulating peripheral veins and arteries (Fig. 10.18).

Thoracocentesis, pericardiocentesis and paracentesis

Anatomy

• Simple fluid collections (e.g. transudate, fresh blood) are hypoechoic (dark) on US (Fig. 10.19) and demonstrate posterior acoustic enhancement.

• Complex collections (e.g. pus, clotted blood) can appear complex and even iso- or hyperechoic (Fig. 10.20). They may contain particles (debris) and even linear structures (e.g. fibrin strands, multi-loculated collections).

• Bowel air and normal lung tissue reflect sound poorly and produce scatter (see Fig. 5.2).

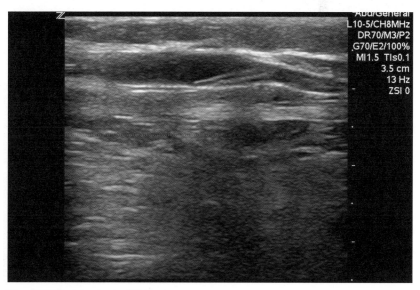

Fig. 10.18 Peripheral vein, US image.

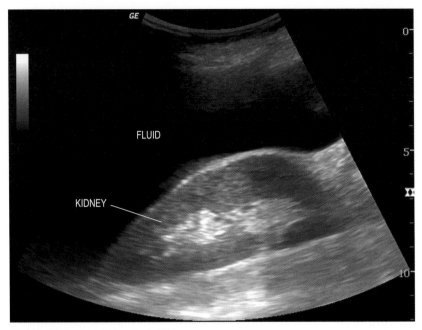

Fig. 10.19 Simple fluid (ascites), US image.

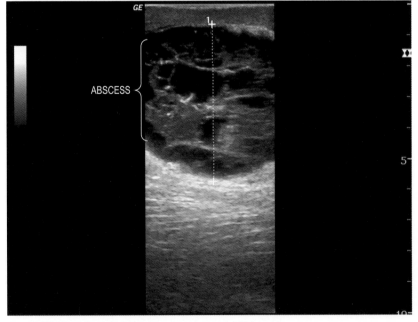

Fig. 10.20 Complex fluid (subcutaneous abscess), US image.

Preparation

- As for CVC (above).
- Specific equipment depends on indication (e.g. whether simple aspiration or insertion of a catheter is required) and local practice (e.g. dedicated pericardiocentesis catheter).
- If sending fluid for analysis: 3-way tap, large syringe, specimen containers.

Patient's position

- This depends on the circumstances. For example, the easiest position for simple aspiration of pleural fluid is patient seated with arms folded, leaning forward, whereas semi-recumbent is preferred for intercostal catheter insertion, and supine for paracentesis (with elevation of the contralateral hip).

Probe and scanner settings

- A curved or even a phased array probe should be used initially to confirm the presence of fluid and nearby anatomical structures. Most operators prefer to switch to a high frequency, linear array probe for a more accurate assessment of depth of the effusion and for real-time guidance, but some prefer to use a curved or phased array probe throughout.
- At least one good view of the fluid should be obtained and recorded.

Probe placement and landmarks

For specific sites, please refer to the following chapters:

- For pleural fluid and pneumothorax, see Ch. 5, *Lung and thorax*.
- For pericardial effusions, see Ch. 6, *Focused echocardiography and volume assessment*.
- For ascites, see Ch. 4, *FAST and EFAST*.

Needle placement

Thoracocentesis

- Identify a site where the effusion is deep, and well above the diaphragm in full expiration.
- If draining a pneumothorax, the recommended site is the fifth intercostal space in the anterior axillary line. An alternative site is the second intercostal space in the mid-clavicular line.
- Insert the needle above a rib to avoid the neurovascular bundle.

Pericardiocentesis

- Traditionally, the subxiphoid approach is taught. However, even a cursory view of the subxiphoid window demonstrates that this approach requires passage of the needle through the liver (see Fig. 6.8).
- Therefore, it is more prudent to approach via the parasternal or apical windows, taking care to avoid the internal thoracic vessels.
- Choose a site where the pericardial effusion is maximal.

Paracentesis

- Traditional teaching has advised needle placement via the left or right iliac fossa, or midline, to avoid the inferior epigastric arteries.
- While US guidance has supplanted this advice to some extent, it is still prudent to ensure that no vessels are inadvertently punctured by the technique. Therefore, avoid excess probe pressure when scanning; otherwise, vessels in the abdominal wall may not be seen.

Handy hints and pitfalls

- ✓ Real-time US guidance of aspiration is safer than merely using US to identify the optimum drainage site for later blind aspiration.
- ✓ If you are not using real-time US but simply using US to mark a needle site before sterilizing the field, do not allow the patient to change position subsequently (e.g. sitting up from supine position). This shifts fluid and organs and mandates that you re-scan the area of interest.
- ✓ Failure to consider diaphragmatic movement with respiration may make these procedures hazardous. So can organomegaly or unusual body habitus.
- ✓ Therefore, always scan through respiration and in at least two planes, paying particular attention to nearby structures, before choosing the optimum site for needle insertion.

- ✓ Before draining fluid, measure the depth of the fluid (Fig. 10.21). This is particularly important to prevent introducing the aspiration needle/cannula too deeply.
- ✓ When no further fluid can be aspirated, re-image the collection to assess its size. If fluid is still present, alter the needle or cannula position to allow further aspiration.
- ✓ When removing a cannula from the thoracic cavity, do so in expiration or during Valsalva manoeuvre to ensure positive intrathoracic pressure.

What US can tell you

- Is there a fluid collection?
- Is it accessible for drainage?
- Is it suitable for drainage? If there is much debris or the collection is multi-loculated, it is probably unsuitable for complete drainage.

What US can't tell you

- The nature of the fluid: e.g. haemothorax, empyema, transudate.

Complications of draining effusions

- Pain.
- Pneumothorax.
- Infection.
- Perforation of nearby organs, e.g. diaphragm, lung, bowel.
- Mistaking fluid within structures such as bladder for ascites.

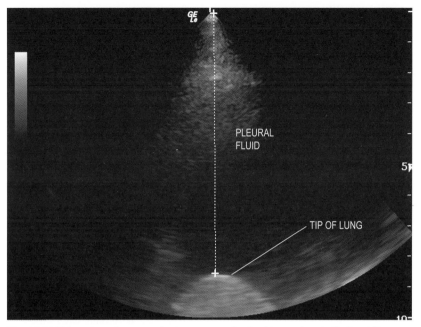

Fig. 10.21 Using phased array probe to measure depth of large pleural effusion, US image.

• Haemorrhage, due to vascular or organ injuries.

Suprapubic catheterization

This is used in the patient in acute retention in whom urethral catheterization is difficult or contraindicated. This may be performed using real-time US guidance (described below) or the site identified using US prior to suprapubic catheter (SPC) insertion.

• Informed consent, dedicated SPC, LA, sterile equipment and sterile US sheath as per local practice.

• Using a low-frequency probe (curved or microconvex), confirm full bladder and identify a site in the midline above the symphysis pubis with no structures overlying the bladder. Mark the site and clean the skin using full aseptic technique.

• Administer LA. While the anaesthetic is taking effect, sterilize the probe and image the bladder again, confirming the optimal site for SPC insertion. (Note: You may continue using the low frequency probe or change to high frequency linear probe depending on body habitus and operator preference.)

• Incise the skin with a scalpel to aid SPC passage. Introduce the SPC and introducer, monitoring progress into the bladder (Fig. 10.22).

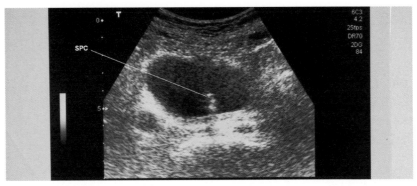

Fig. 10.22 SPC into bladder, US image.

- Observe 'flashback' of urine, remove introducer and secure SPC following manufacturer's instructions.

Lumbar puncture

Although US can visualize deep structures such as the ligamentum flavum in some patients, most operators use it simply to identify the spinous processes of the lumbar vertebrae and to map out the interspinous space for needle entry. Compared with the traditional 'landmark' approach, US-guided lumbar puncture (LP) has a significantly lower failure rate and has been shown to improve the ease of the procedure in obese patients.

Technique

Note: this is a static rather than a real-time technique.
- Informed consent, dedicated LP kit, LA, sterile equipment and sterile US sheath as per usual practice.

Surgical skin marking pen if available.
- Patient position (either lateral foetal or seated, leaning forward) as per blind 'landmark' technique. Palpate landmarks and attempt to identify the line of the spinous processes as usual.
- Using a linear high-frequency probe, scan from right to left with the probe in longitudinal plane until you see the lumbar spinous processes. Like all bony structures, on US they appear bright (echogenic) with posterior acoustic shadows. The midpoint between two such processes is the optimal site for needle placement (Fig. 10.23). Centre this point on the US image then mark the skin on both sides of the middle of the probe (Fig. 10.24). Remove the probe then draw a transverse line connecting the two points.
- Repeat the process in transverse section, identifying the interspinous space and marking the skin on

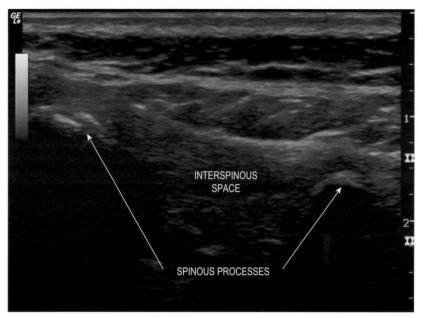

INTERSPINOUS SPACE

SPINOUS PROCESSES

Fig. 10.23 Interspinous space, longitudinal view, US image.

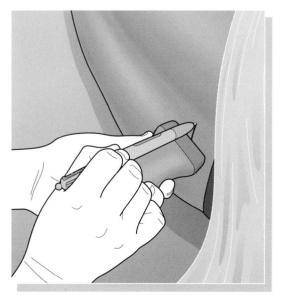

Fig. 10.24 Marking the skin.

Fig. 10.25 Cross drawn on skin.

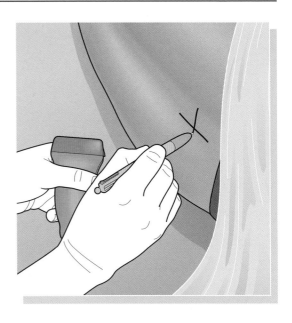

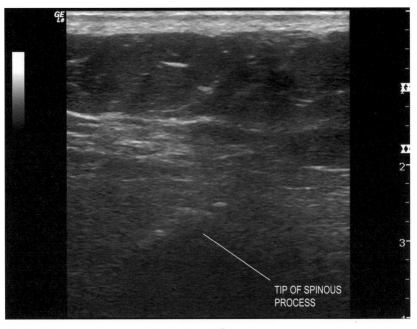

TIP OF SPINOUS PROCESS

Fig. 10.26 Spinous processes, obese patient, US image.

both sides of the middle of the probe. Remove the probe and draw a longitudinal line connecting the two new points until you have a 'cross' or 'X' centred over the site for needle insertion (Fig. 10.25). Prep and drape the site and proceed with LA and LP.

Handy hints and pitfalls

✓ Be very careful to avoid any patient movement between the acts of marking the optimal site and actually inserting the LP needle, otherwise you will need to start again.

✓ Ironically, US is least useful in those patients who require it most for LP, that is the very obese. This is because adipose tissue renders landmarks impalpable and obscures the US image. However, studies have demonstrated that US can identify the pertinent landmarks in 74% of obese patients.

✓ In obese patients the spinous processes may appear simply as ill-defined areas of shadowing (Fig. 10.26).

✓ In the very obese, try an abdominal probe, and alter depth, gain, frequency and greyscale to maximize image quality.

11

Nerve blocks

Justin Bowra, Mike Blaivas

Why use ultrasound?

- By its very nature, regional anaesthesia (peripheral nerve blockade) carries fewer complications than alternatives such as procedural sedation. Common complications include vascular penetration, paraesthesias, haematoma and pneumothorax (when working close to the pleura). Most of these complications are rare even with a traditional blind technique.

- With only a handful of exceptions, peripheral nerve blocks have been the preserve of anaesthetists. This is because of the specialized equipment required (such as nerve stimulators) and the perceived difficulty and unreliability of blind nerve block techniques.

- These difficulties have been overcome with the advent of real-time ultrasound (US) of sufficient image quality to resolve large peripheral nerves. Real-time US can identify the nerve in question and guide the needle to the nerve. US decreases the risk of the complications mentioned above, allows the use of much smaller amounts of local anaesthetic (LA) agent than traditionally used, and assures a higher success rate.

- Nerve stimulators are not required for this technique. This last point is critical for patient comfort. The arm or leg jerking caused by nerve stimulation can be very uncomfortable in the presence of a fracture or other significant injury.

Which blocks?

Real-time US can be used for the following important peripheral nerve blocks (with common indications in parentheses):
- *Upper limb*
  - Interscalene (procedures on upper arm, shoulder). A note of caution: this block is best for the *upper* arm. For example, it commonly misses the medial aspect of the elbow and the hand.
  - Supraclavicular (procedures anywhere on upper limb).

- Infraclavicular (procedures anywhere on upper limb).
- Axillary (procedures on elbow, forearm and hand).
- Median (procedures on lateral palm).
- Ulnar (procedures on medial palm).
- Radial (procedures on dorsum of hand).
- *Lower limb*
  - Femoral (femoral shaft fracture).
  - Sciatic (procedures on back of leg, ankle, foot).
  - Popliteal (procedures on lower leg, ankle, foot).
  - Lateral femoral cutaneous nerve (symptomatic relief of lateral cutaneous nerve syndrome).

US appearance

- Using US, the large roots and trunks of the brachial plexus appear as large hypoechoic rings without a honeycomb appearance, similar to vessels (Fig. 11.1). However, careful observation and Doppler can distinguish these from arteries (which are pulsatile) and veins (which are easily compressible) (Fig. 11.2).
- By contrast, peripheral nerves tend to appear as bright (hyperechoic) tubular bundles of connective tissue, with hypoechoic fascicles (which appear as small dark 'dots' inside the nerve), giving them a heterogeneous 'honeycomb'

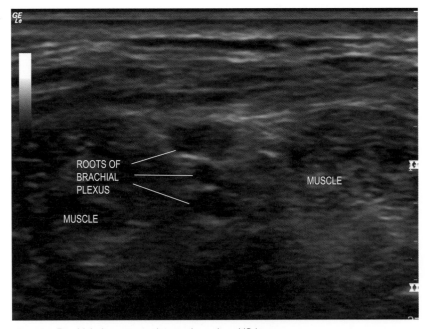

Fig. 11.1 Brachial plexus roots, interscalene view, US image.

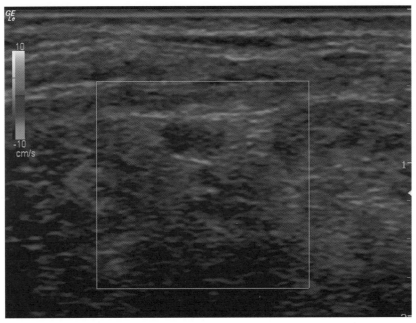

Fig. 11.2 Interscalene view, US Doppler image.

appearance overall. They lie on fascial planes and are usually easy to distinguish from the surrounding muscles, which appear darker (Fig. 11.3).

- In addition, peripheral nerves (unlike the larger roots and trunks) display *anisotropy* on US, which means that their appearance is dependent on the angle of the US beam (Figs 11.3 and 11.4). If the probe is not parallel to the nerve fibres, reflection will not be back towards the probe, and the nerve will appear dark (hypoechoic). To overcome this, carefully scan the same area from different angles.

- Tendons and ligaments can be mistaken for nerves, particularly in transverse section (TS). Like nerves, tendons appear as 'bundles' of echogenic lines on longitudinal scans. Unlike nerves, they do not tend to lie on fascial planes. Also, they are usually brighter (more hyperechoic) than nerves, and in TS their collagen bundles appear as fine dots rather than large circles (Fig. 11.5). If unsure whether a structure is a nerve or tendon, move the distal joint. A tendon will be seen to move separately to the surrounding structures. In addition, tendons exhibit anisotropy more than nerves do.

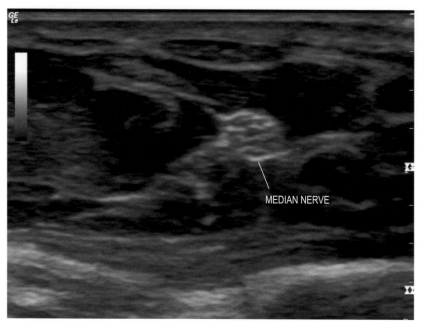

MEDIAN NERVE

Fig. 11.3 Median nerve, honeycomb appearance, US image.

Probe and scanner settings

- High-frequency linear array probe (highest frequency available).
- Multi-beam transducers are critical for a richer and enhanced view of target nerves and are now standard on most machines.
- Nerve preset (musculoskeletal preset is a reasonable alternative).
- Most nerves can be seen with focus depth 3 cm, depth setting 5 cm.

Technique

Screening exam

Before donning sterile gown and gloves, begin with a US 'screening exam' of the area of interest to identify the site and depth of the target nerve and mark the optimum site of needle entry. It is not unheard of to simply be unable to identify the target nerves, and, in such a case, some time and supplies could be saved.

Preparation

- Informed consent unless emergency.
- Patient attached to monitors.
- Resuscitation equipment checked for availability, including intralipid for toxicity. Local anaesthetic, syringe, needle. The exact needle type chosen can vary. For example, anaesthetists often choose non-cutting spinal needles. In general, a large enough bore must be chosen to allow efficient delivery of the LA.

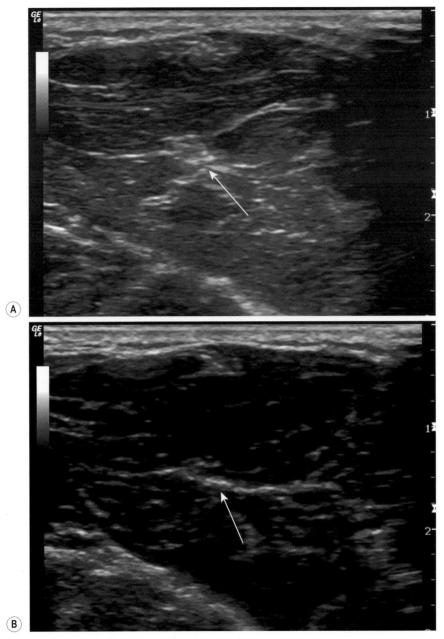

Fig. 11.4 (A), (B) Same site (median nerve) but different probe angle (anisotropy). (B) A slightly different angle of approach renders the entire image darker, including the nerve (arrowed).

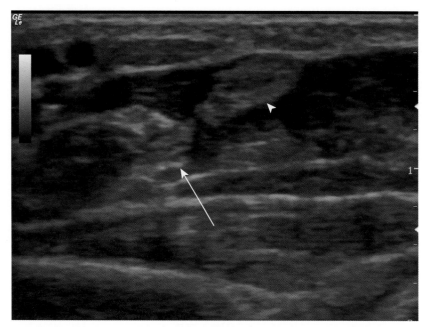

Fig. 11.5 Median nerve (arrowed) and flexor tendon (arrowhead) at wrist, US image.

- US monitor in your line of sight: it is difficult and potentially hazardous to insert a needle when craning to look over your shoulder at the screen. Looking straight up and down will minimize the hand and needle drift that occurs from turning your head. In practice, this often means placing the machine on the other side of the patient from the operator (Fig. 11.6).

Sterile technique

This technique requires a sterile probe and field (see Ch. 10, *Ultrasound-guided procedures*).

TS view of nerve

1. With your non-dominant hand, place probe over the chosen site so that the nerve appears in TS. Identify nerve and nearby structures (e.g. vessels, fascia, muscles) on screen.

2. Move probe and alter image depth and focus so that the nerve appears in the centre of the screen. Optimize the image by adjusting settings including gain. Using colour or power Doppler, make sure the nerves you are looking at are not actually vessels. This is a problem when the nerves are hypoechoic (e.g. interscalene block).

In-plane needle insertion

1. Keep the probe in position with your non-dominant hand.

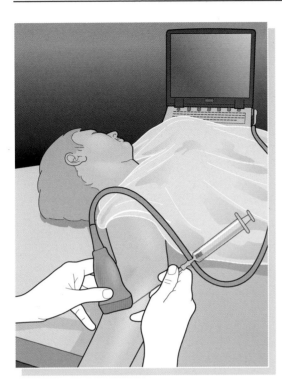

Fig. 11.6 Optimal set-up for median nerve block.

2. With your dominant hand, place the tip of the needle at one end of the probe, so that it is parallel with the long axis of the probe (Figs 11.7 and 11.8). This is known as the *in-plane technique*, and is safer because it allows you to see the whole length of the needle (including its tip) on the screen, rather than the cross-sectional view obtained using a transverse or 'out-of-plane' technique.

3. It is important never to move the transducer and needle at the same time. Dual movement creates disorientation, and it is harder to locate and track your needle.

4. Insert needle at a *shallow angle*. This allows easier visualization of the needle on US (Fig. 11.8). The needle angle can be corrected later. If too shallow an angle is chosen and the needle insertion occurs too far from the target nerve, it is possible to run out of needle. This is best estimated prior to beginning the procedure so the needle does not have to penetrate the skin more than once if possible.

5. The major risk of nerve blocks is inadvertent damage to the nerve or other structures. Avoid this by the following:

Fig. 11.7 Needle position for in-plane technique femoral nerve block.

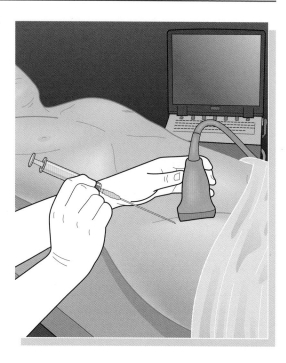

- Choose your needle insertion site away from any nearby vessels. For example, use a lateral approach for femoral nerve block.
- Advance the needle slowly, keeping the *tip* in view on screen at all times. Ensure the plane of the needle parallels the plane of the probe at all times. In general, if the needle is seen the entire time, then inadvertent penetration of sensitive structures should be impossible.
- Stop before the needle reaches the nerve, then infiltrate cautiously. In some cases (such as in the interscalene block),

the nerve bundle sheath has to be penetrated, and this may mean popping the needle through the structure directly adjacent to the nerve. It should be done with care and good visualization of the needle tip.

- Ask the patient to tell you whether he/she feels a sensation of electric shock in the distribution of the nerve. If this occurs, withdraw the needle immediately.

6. Infiltrate LA around the nerve. Watch for the appearance of LA as anechoic (dark) fluid. Infiltrate until the nerve appears to 'float' in the surrounding LA (Fig. 11.9). You will often need to

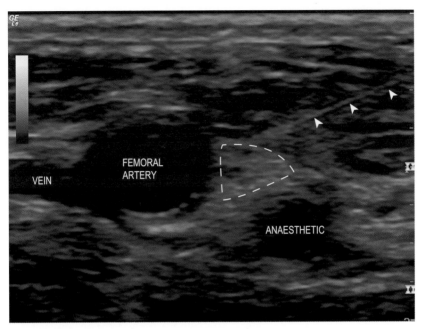

Fig. 11.8 Needle seen (arrowheads) using in-plane technique for femoral nerve block (dashed line), US image.

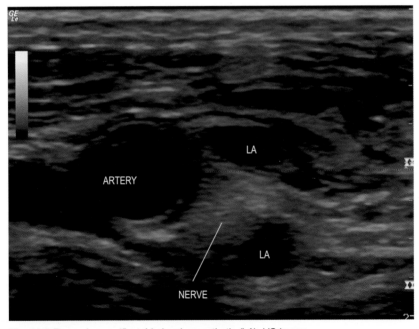

Fig. 11.9 Femoral nerve 'floats' in local anaesthetic (LA), US image.

reposition the needle to achieve this.

7. If working near a vascular structure such as in a femoral nerve block, make sure to aspirate the syringe occasionally to confirm no vascular penetration has occurred.

8. Larger nerves may require larger amounts of LA than smaller ones. This may be especially true for femoral and popliteal nerves.

9. Remove and dispose of the needle.

10. Wait up to 15 minutes (if using long-acting agent such as bupivacaine) and repeat the block if it has been unsuccessful. Full effect may take up to 30 minutes, even though this is likely to apply only to the most distal effects of the block.

Notes on specific nerve blocks

Interscalene block (brachial plexus)

Patient position: supine, head turned away from side of interest. Place probe about halfway down the neck, parallel to the clavicle (Fig. 11.10). Identify the common carotid artery (CCA) and internal jugular vein (IJV) as per central cannulation (see Ch. 10, *Ultrasound-guided procedures*) then slide the probe laterally until you see the anterior and middle scalene muscles. The roots of the brachial plexus appear between these two muscles as three distinct nerve bundles in this location, although individual anatomy may vary (see Fig. 11.1). Slide the probe up and down the neck to find the best view. Confirm the roots are not vessels

Fig. 11.10 Probe placement for interscalene block.

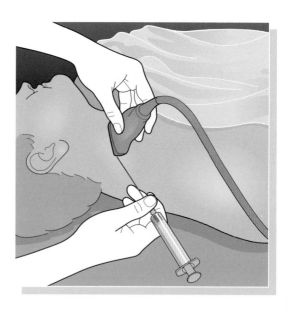

using colour Doppler (see Fig. 11.2). If you can't see the brachial plexus, ask the patient to turn their head and re-scan. This may render the nerve bundles more obvious.

In patients with shoulder dislocation and fractures, lying supine may be very painful, so at times this block has to be performed with the patient recumbent. This position may change the relative anatomy slightly and be confusing to the novice and is best attempted after some experience with the block has been attained. This same rule of thumb applies to the supraclavicular block as well.

Because of the dangers of inadvertently injecting significant structures such as the vertebral artery, epidural space and phrenic nerve blockade, you must be doubly cautious not to advance the needle unless you can see its *tip*.

Supraclavicular block (brachial plexus)

Patient position: supine, head turned away from side of interest. Place probe at the base of the neck in the supraclavicular groove, parallel to the clavicle (Fig. 11.11). Identify the subclavian artery (SA) overlying the first rib. Then identify the smaller, hypoechoic trunks of the brachial plexus lateral to the SA (Fig. 11.12). Note: Although a very effective block,

Fig. 11.11 Probe placement for supraclavicular block.

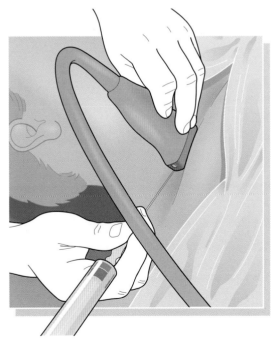

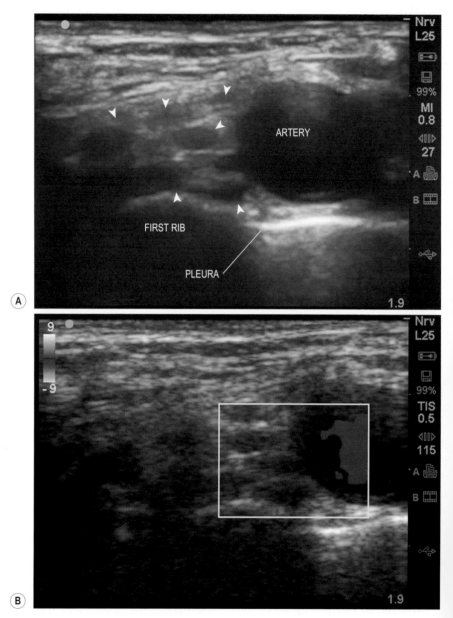

Fig. 11.12 Supraclavicular block view, US images. (A) B-mode: trunks of brachial plexus (arrowed). (B) Doppler image.

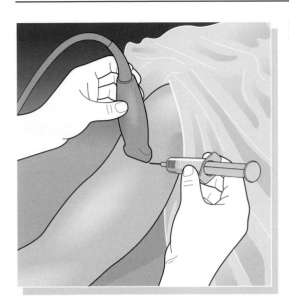

Fig. 11.13 Probe placement for axillary block.

the proximity of the artery and pleura carries a real risk of damage to these important structures.

Axillary block

Patient position: supine, arm turned out exposing the axilla as much as possible. (This block can be performed with the patient partially reclined as well.) Place the probe transversely just inferior to the axilla (Fig. 11.13). The main landmark is the axillary artery in its most proximal location in the upper arm. Scan distally and proximally by a few centimetres for the best view of the nerve. All three nerves targeted by the block at this location sit adjacent to the axillary artery (Fig. 11.14). Infiltrate around each of the three nerves individually. The block works best when coupled with infiltration of the musculocutaneous nerve in the adjacent muscle belly (Figs 11.15 and 11.16).

Median nerve block

Patient position: supine, arm abducted 90 degrees. Place probe transversely on the volar surface of the mid-forearm (Fig. 11.6). Identify the nerve as it runs between the forearm flexor muscles (see Figs 11.3 and 11.4).

Ulnar nerve block

Patient position: supine, arm abducted 90 degrees. Place probe transversely on the volar surface of the distal forearm, near the wrist (Fig. 11.17). Identify the ulnar artery (UA). The ulnar nerve (UN) lies immediately *ulnar* to the UA (Fig. 11.18). Slide the probe proximally, following the nerve until it separates from the artery. The safest possible site for your

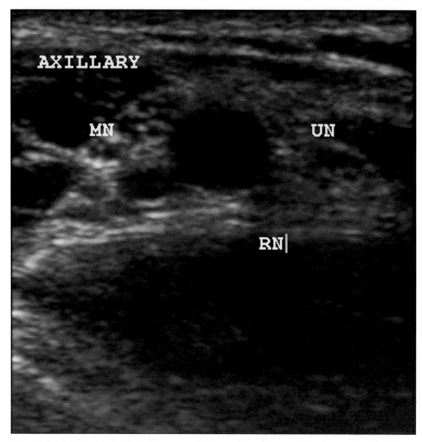

Fig. 11.14 Axillary block view, US image. MN = median nerve; UN = ulnar nerve; RN = radial nerve. Axillary artery is not labelled.

block will be one where the UN is clearly visible and separates from the UA (Fig. 11.19).

Radial nerve block

Patient position: supine, arm abducted 90 degrees. Place probe transversely in the antecubital fossa lateral to the biceps tendon (Fig. 11.20). Identify the nerve between the brachialis and brachioradialis muscles (Fig. 11.21).

Femoral block

Patient position: supine, leg abducted. Place probe at the inguinal crease, parallel to the crease. Here the femoral nerve (FN) is a hyperechoic triangular structure just lateral to the femoral artery, which lies approximately halfway between the symphysis pubis and the anterior superior iliac spine (ASIS). The FN lies deep to the fascia iliaca (see Figs 11.8 and 11.9). The effect of the FN block is

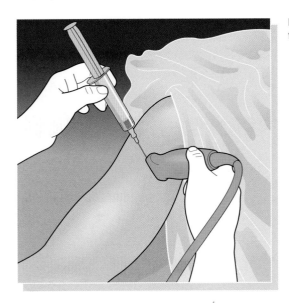

Fig. 11.15 Probe placement for musculocutaneous block.

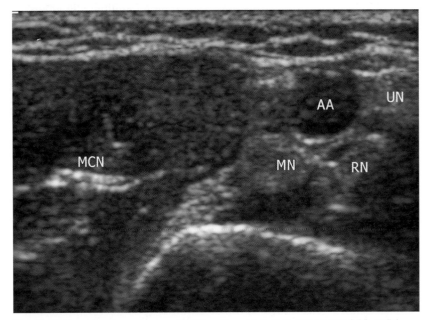

Fig. 11.16 Musculocutaneous nerve (MCN), axillary artery (AA), ulnar nerve (UN), radial nerve (RN), median nerve (MN), US image.

Fig. 11.17 Probe placement for ulnar block.

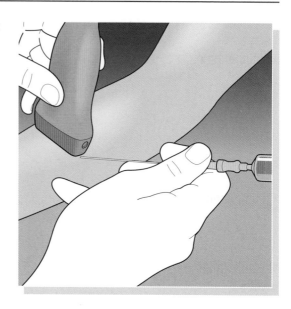

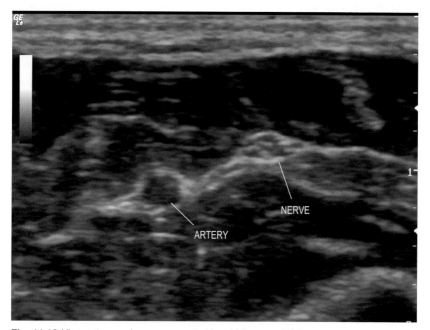

Fig. 11.18 Ulnar artery and nerve separated in mid-forearm, US image.

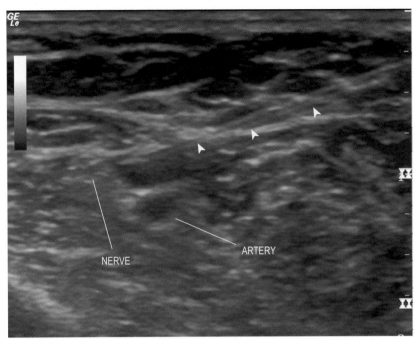

Fig. 11.19 Needle (arrowheads) approaches ulnar nerve, US image.

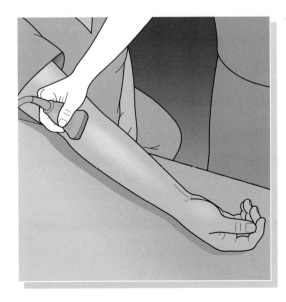

Fig. 11.20 Probe placement for radial block.

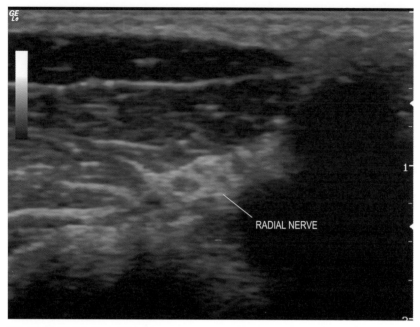

Fig. 11.21 Radial nerve, US image.

optimized by injection of LA within each of the three corners of the triangular femoral nerve formation.

Handy hints and pitfalls

✓ A thorough knowledge of the anatomy and US appearance of nerves is essential, to avoid damaging structures such as tendons.

✓ Because of the potential for significant long-term morbidity, if a major nerve is damaged, exercise caution at all times in nerve blockade, particularly as a novice.

✓ One advantage of the interscalene and axillary blocks over the supraclavicular block is that, if you inadvertently needle a vessel, you can apply direct pressure to stem the bleeding.

✓ Keep the US machine in your line of sight.

✓ Optimize the image with proper settings and gain adjustments.

✓ An assistant is needed to sterilize the probe. If staffing is limited, it is best to rehearse the process beforehand to make sure sterility will be kept.

✓ Measure the required length of needle on the US image before you insert the needle! This will avoid the embarrassment of discovering your needle is too short.

✓ Avoid damaging the nerve or nearby vessels by:

   ✓ Inserting the needle as far away as possible from other structures.

   ✓ Slowing needle insertion, keeping the tip in view at all times.

   ✓ Stopping before the needle reaches the nerve, then infiltrating cautiously.

   ✓ When near vessels, aspirate the syringe to make sure vascular penetration has not accidentally occurred.

   ✓ Withdrawing the needle if patient experiences a sensation of electric shock in the distribution of the nerve.

Summary

➡ Real-time US-guided nerve block is best practice and decreases the risk of complications.

➡ Depending on practice setting, significant nursing time and length of stay, savings may be afforded by avoiding conscious sedation.

➡ The technique can be difficult to learn at first.

   Never puncture what you cannot see. Know what your needle is going through!

12

Deep vein thrombosis

Niall Collum, Russell McLaughlin

The question: is there a deep vein thrombosis?

Deep vein thrombosis (DVT) is the third most common cardiovascular disease in the USA, after acute coronary syndrome and stroke, affecting 2 million individuals per annum. The annual incidence of DVT in the UK is 0.5–1 per 1000 adults, i.e. up to 60 000 cases per annum. Pulmonary embolism (PE) is recognized as the cause of death in approximately 8000 people per annum in the UK, and 90% of PE have DVT as the source. In reality, the incidence of both PE and DVT is probably much higher due to significant under-diagnosis.

Many patients will present themselves, or be referred by their general practitioner, to the emergency department (ED) for investigation with a painful or swollen leg. Clinical examination for DVT is unreliable, and further investigation is often required.

It is crucial that the diagnosis of DVT be made early and accurately, allowing treatment to be instituted at an early stage.

Why use compression ultrasound?

Compression ultrasound (US) has become the diagnostic modality of choice by radiologists for symptomatic DVT with both sensitivity and specificity of 98–100% reported for proximal DVT. In addition, compression US in the ED has been shown to reduce significantly the time to diagnosis for this group of patients.

Three-point compression US is a simplification of standard compression US that is easily learned, rapid to perform, and has been shown to be highly accurate in the diagnosis of proximal DVT. Sensitivity of 93–100% and specificity of 97–100% for proximal DVT is reported. Benefits include diagnosis at point of care, streamlined patient flow and decreased demand upon radiology departmental services.

A limitation of three-point compression US is missed isolated *below-knee* DVT. However, many clinicians consider that in patients with isolated below-knee DVT, the drawbacks of anticoagulation (risk of complications, cost and inconvenience) may exceed the benefits.

In DVT the major health risks are propagation and/or embolization. The risk of embolization in a patient who may have *below-knee* DVT, but with no evidence of proximal DVT on compression US, is quoted as between 0.7% and 1.1%. However, the risk of propagation of below-knee DVT is quoted as ranging from 2% to 36%. Patients, therefore, who have normal three-point compression testing, but who are at high risk for DVT as defined by a validated clinical assessment tool, should have a repeat scan at approximately 1 week. Local treatment protocols should be followed as regards indication for anticoagulation during this period.

An example of a clinical risk assessment tool (Wells' criteria) is given in Table 12.1.

Anatomy (Fig. 12.1)

- The popliteal vein begins as the confluence of the calf veins behind the knee. It lies superficial to the popliteal artery in the popliteal fossa and ascends to the adductor canal where it becomes the femoral vein (also known as the superficial femoral vein).

- The femoral vein is found anteromedially in the thigh: initially deep to the femoral artery, coming to lie more medially as it ascends. The profunda femoris vein joins the femoral vein approximately 4 cm below the inguinal ligament, becoming the common femoral vein.

- The long saphenous vein joins just proximal to the common femoral vein. The common femoral vein becomes the external iliac vein as

Table 12.1 Wells' criteria: a clinical risk assessment tool	
Clinical parameter	**Score**
Active cancer (treatment ongoing, or within 6 months or palliative)	+1
Paralysis or recent plaster immobilization of the lower extremities	+1
Recently bedridden for >3 days or major surgery <4 weeks	+1
Localized tenderness along the distribution of the deep venous system	+1
Entire leg swelling	+1
Calf swelling >3 cm compared to the asymptomatic leg	+1
Pitting oedema (greater in the symptomatic leg)	+1
Previous DVT documented	+1
Collateral superficial veins (non-varicose)	+1
Alternative diagnosis (as likely or greater than that of DVT)	−2
Total of above score	
High probability of DVT	2 or more
Low probability	less than 2
DVT = deep vein thrombosis.	

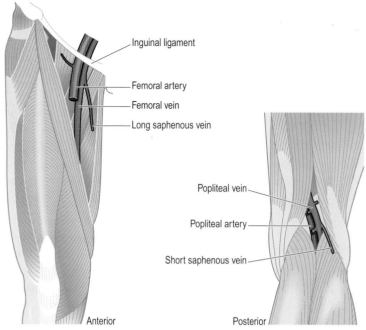

Fig. 12.1 Relations of the femoral and popliteal veins.

it passes superiorly, under the inguinal ligament.

Clinical picture

This is often unreliable. If in doubt, assume that the patient has DVT until proven otherwise.

- The history: classically, a history of atraumatic calf or thigh pain and swelling, with recognized risk factors such as immobilization, recent surgery, smoking and active cancer.
- The examination: classically leg swelling, calf tenderness along the distribution of the deep veins, pitting oedema in the symptomatic leg and absence of a likely alternative diagnosis.

- Associated symptoms/signs of PE may be present: breathlessness; pleuritic chest pain; collapse; tachycardia; tachypnoea; hypotension.
- Bear in mind that there is a broad differential diagnosis: for example, symptomatic Baker's cyst, cellulitis, superficial thrombophlebitis, soft-tissue injury, lymphadenopathy.

 If in doubt, assume that the patient has DVT until proven otherwise.

Before you scan

- Ensure that the area to be used is private.

- Darkened room.
- Ensure that the patient is comfortable.
- Have an adequate supply of US gel.

The technique and views

Patient's position

Groin to adductor canal (Fig. 12.2)

- Supine, with acoustic jelly along the course of the femoral vein.
- Leg abducted to 10–15 degrees, slight external rotation.

Popliteal segment (Fig. 12.3)

- Partial decubitus, affected leg uppermost.
- Or seated with knee flexed and lower leg hanging over the side of the examination table.
- Knee flexed to 25–30 degrees (removes tension on popliteal fascia and vein).

Probe and scanner settings

- Standard B-mode soft tissue settings.
- Linear transducer, high-frequency (5.0–7.5 MHz); a low-frequency probe may be required in larger patients.
- Depth setting 3–4 cm.
- Focus depth 3 cm.

Probe placement and landmarks

- Hold the probe in transverse position throughout, with the probe marker to the patient's right (see Fig. 12.2). (If trying to compress veins in the longitudinal position, the probe may 'slip off' and give a false impression of compression.)
- Start in groin just below the mid-point of the inguinal ligament. Rest the probe lightly on the skin,

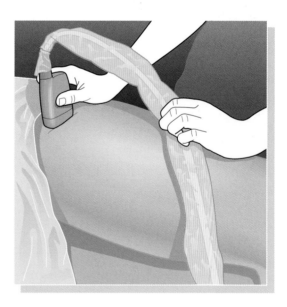

Fig. 12.2 Initial patient position (supine) with probe at groin.

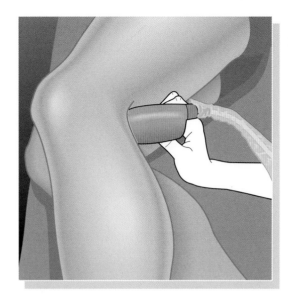

Fig. 12.3 Next patient position (partial decubitus) with probe in popliteal fossa.

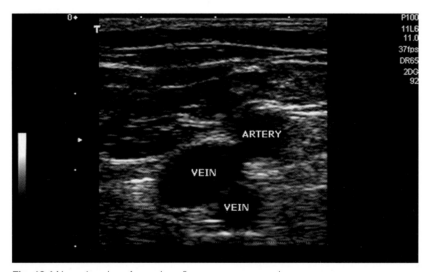

Fig. 12.4 Normal saphenofemoral confluence, no compression.

identifying the 'Mickey Mouse' sign (Fig. 12.4):

- Femoral artery (thick-walled) seen pulsating lateral to femoral vein

- Saphenofemoral venous confluence: thinner-walled, transmitted pulsation only.

- Gentle compression will appose the anterior and posterior walls of

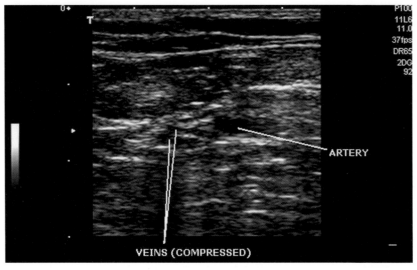

ARTERY

VEINS (COMPRESSED)

Fig. 12.5 Normal saphenofemoral confluence, compression.

normal veins; arteries are relatively incompressible.

- Place the probe in the optimum position for saphenofemoral confluence. Record and save copies of two views: one without compression, one with compression, apposing the vein walls (Figs 12.4 and 12.5).

- Follow the femoral vein distally compressing and releasing, ideally until the entire length has been visualized to the adductor hiatus (see 'Handy hints', below). Record and save two views (Figs 12.6 and 12.7).

- Re-position the patient as described above, to evaluate the popliteal segment.

- With the probe in the popliteal fossa, identify the popliteal vein lying superficially, with the artery pulsating deeply to this.

- Follow the popliteal vein superiorly to the adductor hiatus and inferiorly to the confluence of the calf veins, compressing and releasing. Record and save two views (Figs 12.8 and 12.9).

If at any point the vein is seen to have echogenic material within the lumen, and/or is found to be incompressible, then the patient has a DVT at this site. The examination can be terminated at this point (Figs 12.10 and 12.11).

Essential views

A minimum of six views must be obtained on the leg of interest:

- saphenofemoral confluence with and without compression
- distal femoral vein with and without compression
- popliteal vein with and without compression.

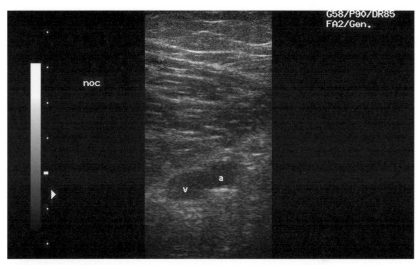

Fig. 12.6 Normal distal thigh; no compression (noc). v = vein; a = artery.

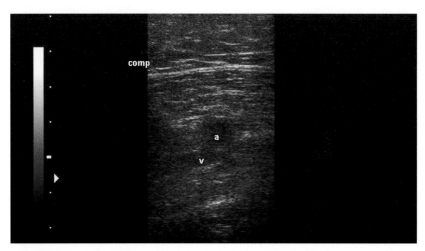

Fig. 12.7 Normal distal thigh, compression (comp). v = vein; a = artery.

All views should be clearly labelled with anatomical site, whether compression applied, and artery and veins identified.

Handy hints

✓ Strictly speaking, three-point compression US requires that only

the groin, mid-thigh and popliteal fossa be scanned, because veins distal to a DVT usually are minimally compressible to non-compressible. However, a common sense approach is to scan as much of the femoral vein as possible.

✓ Use plenty of gel.

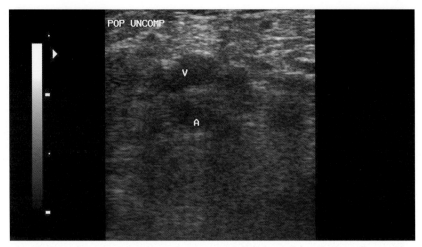

Fig. 12.8 Normal popliteal, no compression. V = vein; A = artery.

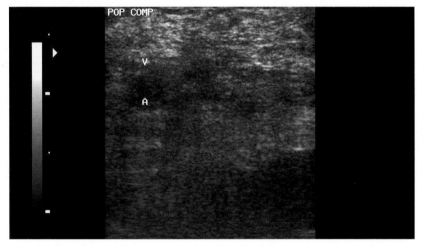

Fig. 12.9 Normal popliteal, compression. V = vein; A = artery.

✓ Press lightly to avoid obliterating the venous lumen (particularly in the popliteal fossa).

✓ A Valsalva manoeuvre may help to identify the femoral vein if there is any doubt. The normal response is a 15% increase in venous diameter on straining. (This also assists in exclusion of occlusive thrombus in the iliac veins; however, the response will be less marked in a patient with congestive cardiac failure (CCF).)

✓ The use of colour flow and/or pulse wave Doppler may assist with differentiation of the femoral vein

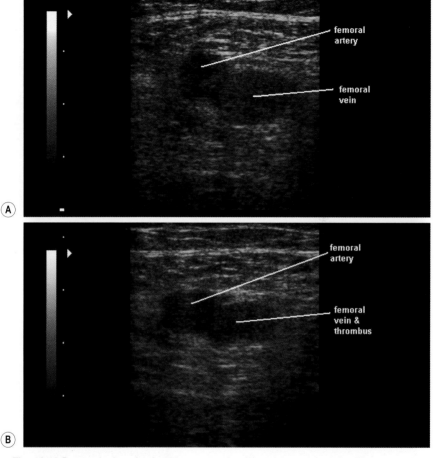

femoral
artery

femoral
vein

femoral
artery

femoral
vein &
thrombus

(A)

(B)

Fig. 12.10 Deep vein thrombosis with compression (A) and no compression (B).

and artery, although this is not usually necessary. (Fig. 12.12).

✓ When progressing down the thigh, depth of field and focal depth may need to be increased.

✓ In obese patients, it may be necessary to use the lower-frequency (abdominal) probe, as the high-frequency probe loses resolution at depth.

✓ If the popliteal vein cannot be seen easily in the decubitus position, then scan the vein again with the patient seated or standing up.

✓ Patients with previous venous disease including DVT may have incompressible veins, resulting in a false-positive result.

✓ Up to 35% of the population have duplex popliteal veins. Ensure that

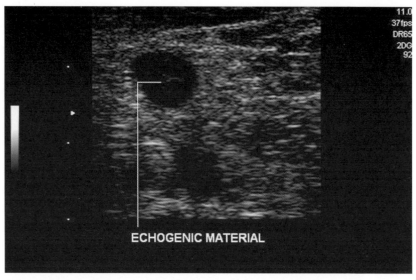

Fig. 12.11 Deep vein thrombosis; note intraluminal echogenic material.

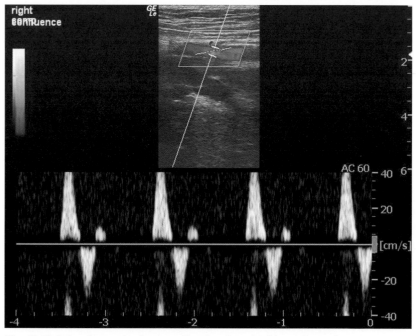

Fig. 12.12 Colour flow and pulse wave Doppler of proximal femoral vessels.

this segment particularly is well visualized, to avoid false-negative results.

✓ If any segment cannot be adequately visualized, then call the study inadequate and refer to the radiology department.

What three-point compression US can tell you

• The presence or absence of proximal DVT; i.e. popliteal vein and above.

What three-point compression US can't tell you

• Presence or absence of *calf* vein DVT.
• The likelihood of propagation or thromboembolism.
• The cause of the pain if US is normal.

Now what?

• Proximal DVT: treat as per local treatment protocols.
• No proximal DVT:
  • Patients with a high risk of *below-knee* DVT and normal proximal veins should probably be re-scanned at 48 hours to 1 week to rule out propagation of DVT.
  • Other patients should be reassessed for other causes of their presentation.
• Inadequate scan: refer to radiology and consider treatment for DVT in the interim period.

Summary

➡ Three-point compression US is a useful investigation, which can diagnose proximal DVT quickly and accurately.
➡ This timely diagnosis can improve patient flow in both the emergency and radiology departments.

13

Musculoskeletal and soft tissues

Niall Collum, Russell McLaughlin

The questions

- Is there an effusion?
- Is there an abscess?
- Is there a dislocation?
- Is there a fracture?

Paediatric hip effusion

Atraumatic hip pain is a common presenting symptom in children and can be caused by a number of inflammatory and infectious diseases. The limping child may have pathology in a variety of anatomical sites, and it may be difficult to pinpoint this site by clinical and X-ray assessment alone. The use of bedside ultrasound (US) to rapidly identify a hip effusion as the cause is of benefit in reducing the differential diagnoses, and may avoid unnecessary treatments such as plastering for suspected toddler's fracture.

Atraumatic hip pain is much less common in adults and the hip joint is correspondingly harder to image. The principles outlined in this chapter may be extrapolated to adult hip scanning, indeed to the diagnosis and treatment of effusions in most joints.

Why use US?

- *Diagnosis.* US uses no ionizing radiation, is cheap and takes only minutes to perform. Accurate reproducible measurements of effusion size are possible. Older children think that this is a 'cool' test—no needles!
- *Localization and drainage.* US can be used to guide aspiration of the effusion.
- *Other joints.* Although clinical identification and aspiration via the landmark technique is sufficient for large effusions in other joints (e.g. knee), US localization is useful for small effusions and in the obese.

Clinical picture

The child with a painful hip usually presents with a limp. There may be associated pyrexia. It is sometimes difficult to be sure which side is affected and rarely the presentation will be bilateral. A variety of conditions cause atraumatic hip pain in paediatric patients including:

- transient synovitis
- septic arthritis
- Perthes' disease
- slipped capital femoral epiphysis (SCFE).

Before you scan

- Explain to the child and parents the need for the procedure and obtain informed consent.
- Place the patient supine on a couch.
- Distraction techniques for the young child may be helpful. Involve the parents/guardians if possible. Dimmed background lighting is desirable. Perhaps the child could hold the probe for a few moments at the start to reassure them. (Don't let them drop it!)

- Exposure of the hip area is necessary, but the undergarment/nappy should usually be retained.

The technique and views

Patient's position

- Ideal: supine with hips in the neutral position without flexion (Fig. 13.1).
- However, it is more important to keep the child still than to obtain positioning perfection. If the child is reluctant to straighten the hip fully, ensure that both hips are examined in exactly the same position.
- This is a completely different technique from that used to identify developmental dysplasia of hip. This can cause confusion.

Fig. 13.1 Patient supine, probe parallel to long-axis femoral neck.

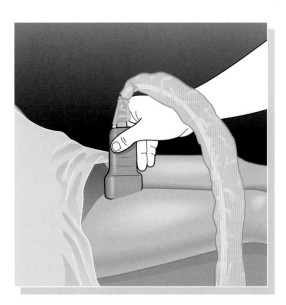

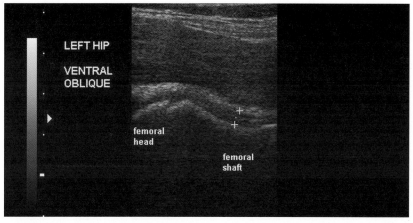

Fig. 13.2 Normal hip joint, ventral oblique view, landmarks labelled, measurement calipers in situ.

 Both hips must be examined in the same position with the legs as straight as is comfortable.

Probe and scanner settings

1. High-frequency (7–12 MHz) linear array probe.

2. Many scanners will have a paediatric hip/musculoskeletal preset. If not, use up to three focal spots set with the deepest spot just on the bone surface, usually a few centimetres deep.

3. Optimize the gain and grey map so that the soft tissues are relatively dark to allow visualization of a 'black' effusion.

Probe placement and landmarks

1. Scan the hip anteriorly in an oblique plane along the long axis of the femoral neck (Fig. 13.1).

2. You should be able to identify (Fig. 13.2):
   - the brightly echogenic cortex of the femoral head and neck
   - the anterior margin of the acetabulum
   - the echolucent physis (growth plate)
   - the iliopsoas muscle superficial to the joint capsule
   - the anterior recess of the normal joint capsule, its anterior and posterior margins parallel ('tram tracking')
   - the normal capsule has a *concave contour* and the distance from its outer margin to the cortex of the femoral neck measures 2–5 mm.

3. Measure at the widest point at 90 degrees to the bony cortex using electronic calipers (Fig. 13.2).

4. Compare the two sides. The hip capsules' depths should be

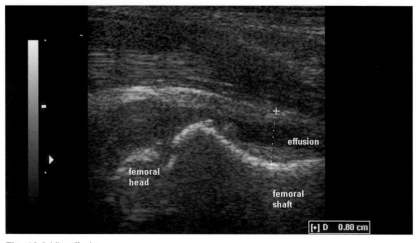

Fig. 13.3 Hip effusion.

symmetric to within 2 mm of each other.

5. Pathology. When there is an effusion, one or more of the following will be observed (Fig. 13.3):

- Anechoic fluid distends capsule: convex margin, loss of 'tram tracking'.
- Capsule depth greater than 5 mm.
- Asymmetry: the affected joint's capsular depth will be more than 2 mm deeper than the normal side.

Note: In infants, clearly the upper limit of normal capsule depth will be less than 5 mm. In such cases, convexity and asymmetry are used as indicators of effusion.

Septic joints may contain echogenic debris, but some septic joints will be clear and many joints with debris are not infected. This is *not* a reliable sign.

Arthrocentesis

Not all effusions require aspiration. Decision to aspirate depends on the clinical picture and other investigations (see below, 'Now what?'). Joint aspiration can be performed in the emergency department (ED), operating theatre (OT) or in the radiology department depending on the patient and local practice.

If aspirating the joint, you will require:

- Explanation and informed consent.
- A co-operative patient: this may entail local anaesthetic and/or conscious sedation (with appropriate medical assistance and monitoring) or even general anaesthetic in the OT.

- Sterile technique, sterile US probe sheath and gel (see also Ch. 10, *Ultrasound-guided procedures*).
- suitable needle and syringe
- specimen jars for laboratory analysis of the fluid.

The technique of US-guided hip-joint aspiration is similar to that used for draining effusions (Ch. 10, *Ultrasound-guided procedures*). Introduce the needle along the long axis of the probe. Identify the needle (and/or its ring-down artefact) on the US image, monitoring the needle's progress into the collection and aspirate.

Essential views

One view of each hip identically positioned (in practice take three of each and use the best one).

Handy hints

✓ Compare both sides (Fig. 13.4). Scan the asymptomatic side first to gain the child's trust.

✓ Beware bilateral joint effusion.

✓ Measure depth perpendicular to the *cortex*. Measurement at an angle will overestimate depth (Fig. 13.5).

What US can tell you

- Is there an effusion? US accuracy is >90%.

What US can't tell you

- The cause of the effusion. Occasionally the 'slip' of an SCFE

may be seen or fragmentation of the femoral head in Perthes' disease. These, however, are late signs and their absence is not helpful. If fluid analysis is required, needle aspiration must be carried out. However, US is useful when analysed together with clinical findings and other investigations such as white cell count.

- Is there an infection? A negative scan makes septic arthritis very unlikely but does not exclude *osteomyelitis*.

Now what?

- No effusion on US: look for other cause of presentation.
- Inadequate scan: repeat and reassess patient.
- Effusion on US: further investigations (e.g. blood tests, plain X-ray, magnetic resonance imaging) and management depend on clinical features and local practice.
- Aspiration of the effusion is often unnecessary: for example, in a child with a clinical and laboratory picture of improving transient synovitis.
- Joint aspiration can be performed in the ED, OT or in the radiology department depending on the patient and local practice.

 Not all hip effusions require aspiration.

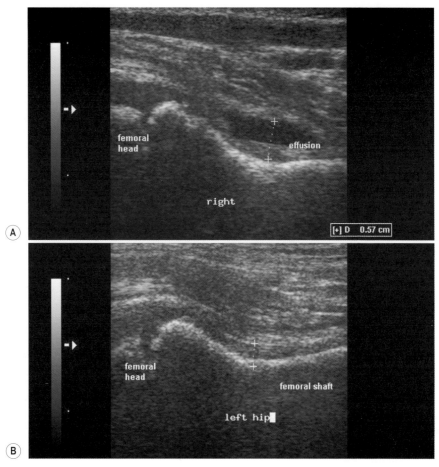

Fig. 13.4 Comparative views. Affected hip (A) is >2 mm wider than normal side (B).

Summary

- US can quickly, safely and reliably identify hip effusions.
- A single adequate view of each hip is all that is required.
- The identification or exclusion of an effusion helps guide patient management.
- US can be used to guide joint aspiration.
- US does not tell you the cause of the effusion.

Soft tissue infections

Cellulitis is a common reason for presentation to EDs, with a reported 70 000 hospital episodes per annum in the UK. Abscess formation is a recognized complication which may be clinically occult. Any improvement in diagnostic accuracy should bring clinical benefit, as its

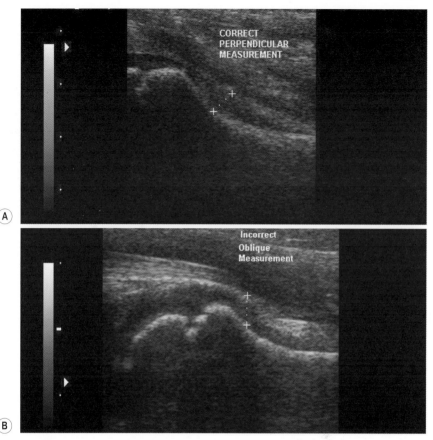

Fig. 13.5 (A) Correct depth measurement (perpendicular to cortex), (B) incorrect (angled) measurement.

management differs significantly from cellulitis. With rising community-acquired methicillin-resistant *Staphylococcus aureus* (MRSA) soft tissue infections, which have a high incidence of abscess formation, the need to differentiate between the two is more important than ever.

Why use US?

- US enables the presence or absence of fluid collection to be identified rapidly.
- US by emergency physician has been shown to improve the accuracy of diagnosis of subcutaneous abscess.

- US may enable more accurate use of aspiration or incision and drainage, reducing unnecessary procedures.

The technique and views

- Position the patient comfortably, with the affected area exposed.
- Provide analgesia consistent with good clinical practice.
- Use the high-frequency (7– 12 MHz) linear array probe.
- Scan the entire area of clinical concern dynamically in two planes, printing/saving several images as you go.
- Alter the gain so that fluid in nearby blood vessels *just* appears black. If gain is set too dark, then tissues such as fat and muscle can appear black to the novice and lead to incorrect diagnosis of abscess where none exists. This can be embarrassing when inserting a needle.

If aspiration is to be performed:
- Ensure patient is appropriately consented and prepared.
- Provide topical, regional or sedation/general anaesthesia as appropriate.
- Sterile technique, sterile US probe sheath and gel.
- Use the probe and needle 'in plane', i.e. with the needle and the probe scan plane parallel, enabling visualization of the needle throughout its length.

- Follow the needle image as it is directed towards the collection, and aspirate when the tip is seen to enter the collection.

Normal anatomy

It is important to interpret US images within an applied anatomical knowledge context. Bone appears as an echobright structure with posterior shadowing, while muscle appears relatively dark with 'marbling'. Fascial planes are identified as relatively echogenic lines, and subcutaneous tissue has a relatively brightly speckled appearance (Fig. 13.6).

US appearances of pathology

Cellulitis and abscess can be reliably differentiated using US, although it must be borne in mind that the clinical and US appearances only represent a snapshot of a dynamic disease process. Repeated clinical/US review may be warranted.

In early cellulitis, US appearances may be normal, or exhibit only a subtle increase in echogenicity.

As cellulitis progresses, hypoechogenic stranding occurs in subcutaneous tissues, conferring a reticular pattern which has been described as 'cobblestoning'. This is US evidence of subcutaneous oedema and inflammatory change. It generally precedes abscess formation (Fig. 13.7).

Abscess formation is identified as a well-defined hypoechoic area which displaces the normal tissue

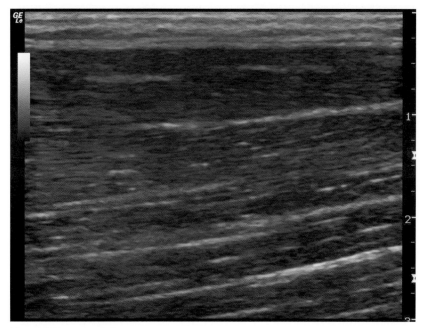

Fig. 13.6 Normal soft tissue.

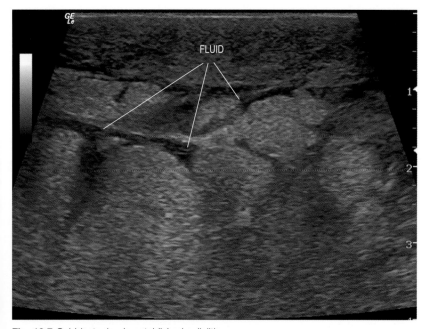

Fig. 13.7 Cobblestoning in established cellulitis.

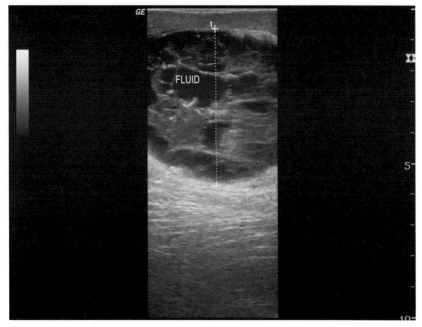

Fig. 13.8 Loculated abscess with posterior enhancement.

architecture (Fig. 13.8). Debris is often visible in this hypoechoic area, and some minor movement of this fluid may be noted.

Posterior enhancement artefact may also be noted.

What US can tell you

- Is there a fluid collection/abscess?
- Relationship to local anatomical structures.
- Guide to aspiration.

What US can't tell you

- The likelihood of successful aspiration versus need for incision and drainage.

Summary

- ➡ US can quickly, safely and reliably identify abscess.
- ➡ US can assist in clinical decision-making.
- ➡ US can be used to guide abscess drainage in real time.

Shoulder dislocation

Shoulder dislocation accounts for approximately 50% of all joint dislocations, affecting between 1% and 2% of the population. Between 90% and 98% of these are anterior dislocations, and there is a high recurrence rate (≥50%) if managed conservatively.

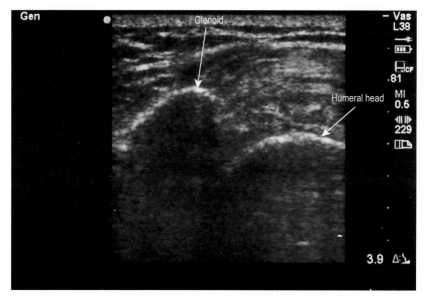

Fig. 13.9 Posterolateral view of shoulder showing normal bony configuration.

Why use US?

- Clinical confirmation of dislocation and reduction may be challenging in the muscular or the obese.
- US can rapidly confirm the presence of dislocation at the bedside.
- US can also confirm successful reduction at the bedside.
- It may be possible to significantly reduce the cumulative radiation doses in select patient groups (e.g. recurrent/habitual dislocators).

Anatomy

The shoulder joint may be scanned anteriorly, superiorly or posteriorly. We strongly recommend a posterior view for the recognition of dislocation and reduction. The authors are convinced that this position is the easiest one to recognize abnormal anatomy in dislocated shoulders, and enables reduction to be easily visualized.

This position enables the clinician to avoid the acromioclavicular arch superiorly, and the coracoid process anteriorly. It also enables the posterior aspect of the glenoid rim to be easily identified (Fig. 13.9).

The technique and views

- Position the patient comfortably, with the shoulder area exposed posterosuperiorly.
- Provide adequate analgesia.
- Use the high-frequency (7– 12 MHz) linear array probe.
- The probe position is transverse, placed on the posterosuperior

shoulder, with the marker directed laterally.

- Depth of field is usually between 3 and 7 cm, dependent upon body habitus.

US appearances

When visualized in the plane described above, the normal glenoid rim and the humeral head should be easily identified as echogenic structures; with posterior shadowing, equidistant from the skin surface (Fig. 13.9).

Anterior dislocation is identified by a disruption of this normal relationship, whereby the glenoid labrum is identified at a normal depth, but the humeral head is visible deeper in the field of view (i.e. displaced and lying further anteriorly) (Fig. 13.10).

Essential views

- Pre-reduction (Fig. 13.10).
- Post-reduction (Fig. 13.9), i.e. normal anatomical configuration.

Handy hints

✓ If doubt exists re the view, scan both sides for comparison.

✓ When reduction is successful, the humeral head can be gently internally and externally rotated under direct vision using US.

✓ US should not replace plain X-ray in the assessment of the shoulder for associated fracture.

What US can tell you

- Presence of dislocation and reduction.

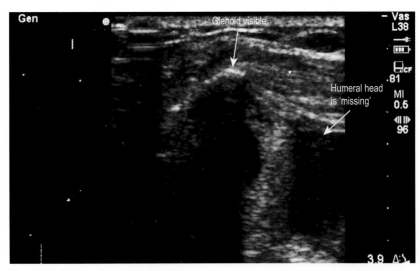

Fig. 13.10 Anterior dislocation, humeral head is so deep to glenoid it is in fact 'missing'.

What US can't tell you

- Absence of associated subtle fracture.

Summary

➡ US can confirm dislocation and reduction.
➡ US may reduce the use of plain X-ray, specifically pre-reduction films.
➡ US does not replace plain X-ray.

Fracture diagnosis

The diagnosis and management of trauma is a core skill in emergency medicine. Plain X-ray is the modality used to identify most fractures, but other modalities including US, CT and MRI are possible alternatives. There is evidence for the superiority of US over plain X-ray in the diagnosis of sternal and rib fracture, and US has been proposed as an accurate and viable alternative to X-ray in the diagnosis of paediatric forearm fractures. US may be particularly valuable in the diagnosis of fracture in resource-limited settings.

Why use US?

- It is a rapid, relatively painless (if applied gently), bedside test.
- US involves no ionizing radiation.
- US may have a particular role for selected fracture types.

The technique and views (distal radius and ulna)

- Position the patient comfortably, with the forearm exposed.
- Provide adequate analgesia.
- Use the high-frequency (7–12 MHz) linear array probe.
- The depth of field is usually less than 5 cm.
- The probe should be used longitudinally along the limb, and imaged dynamically.
- Six planes of view should be obtained:
  - Volar, dorsal and radial aspects of the radius (Fig. 13.11A–C).
  - Volar, dorsal and ulnar aspects of the ulna (Fig. 13.12A,B).

US appearances

The echogenic bony cortices are easy to identify, with posterior shadowing and overlying normal soft tissue appearances (Fig. 13.12).

Fractures may be recognized by three key US features:
- A subtle break in the echogenic cortex (Fig. 13.13).
- An angulation in the cortex (Fig. 13.14).
- An echo-poor (dark) area corresponding to the haematoma.

Handy hints

✓ Scan systematically as described above, but focus on the area of tenderness.

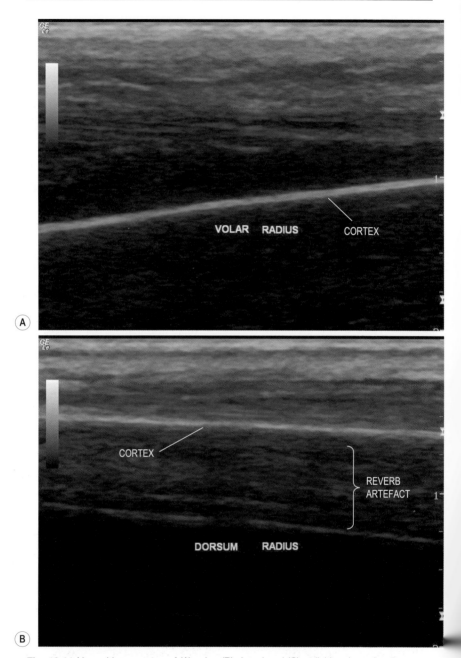

Fig. 13.11 Normal bony cortex of (A) volar, (B) dorsal and (C) radial borders of radius.

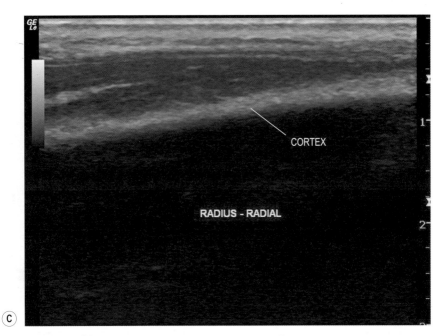

Fig. 13.11 cont'd.

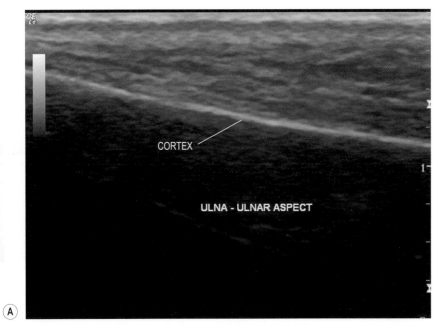

Fig. 13.12 Normal bony cortex of (A) ulnar, (B) dorsal borders of ulna.

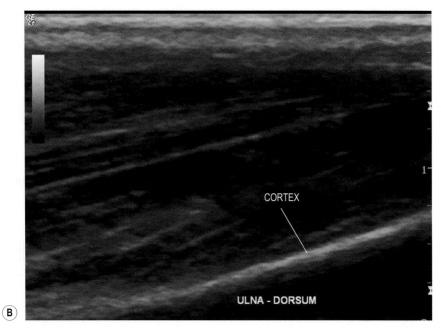

Fig. 13.12 cont'd.

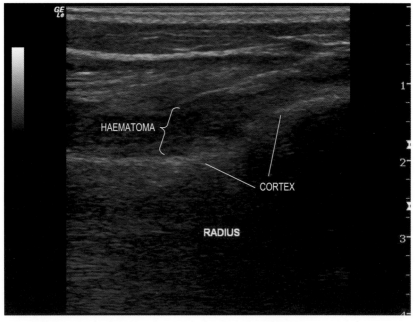

Fig. 13.13 Cortical break and associated echo-poor haematoma.

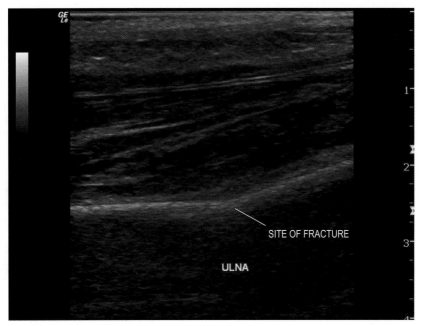

SITE OF FRACTURE

ULNA

Fig. 13.14 Angulation of cortex.

✓ However, scan as gently as possible. After all, the alternative to US is a painless X-ray, whereas pressure from the US probe on a fracture can easily hurt a child.

What US can tell you

• Presence or absence of fracture.
• In some instances cortical alignment can be assessed post reduction.

What US can't tell you

• Conformation of that fracture (e.g. comminution, articular involvement).

Summary

➡ US has proven accuracy in the diagnosis of some fractures, e.g. sternal/rib, distal radial.
➡ US has the potential to reduce the use of plain X-ray.
➡ US has not yet been shown to be sensitive enough to replace plain X-ray in limb trauma.
➡ US is not a useful modality to confirm or rule out associated shoulder fracture.

14 Soft-tissue foreign bodies

Russell McLaughlin

The question: is there a foreign body?

To answer this question one must first employ the basic principles of history and examination followed by investigation. The question may be answered at any stage in this process. However, a foreign body (FB) can be missed at any stage in this process and no single emergency department (ED) investigation is universally applicable. Do not stray from the binary question: 'FB: Yes or No?'.

Why use ultrasound?

Ultrasound (US) is extremely useful for identifying or excluding soft-tissue FBs not readily visible on X-ray. Examples include wood, plastic or aluminium. Even if an FB is visible on plain X-ray, the dynamic nature of US is a far superior aid to FB removal.

Clinical picture

The patient can usually detail the injury and describe the suspected FB and how it entered the skin. History may not be complete in certain situations (e.g. in paediatric and delayed presentations or if intoxication has been a contributing factor). Despite negative investigations, a patient complaining of persisting FB sensation or ongoing wound infection (persistent discharge, sinus formation or poor healing) should be assumed to have an FB until proven otherwise.

The technique and views

Patient's position

- Dictated by clinical picture.
- FB in hand/forearm: seated, resting both forearms on examination couch.
- FB torso/lower limb: supine or prone.

Probe and scanner settings

- Superficial FB: high-frequency probe (10–15 MHz) with a thick layer of sterile transducer gel.
- Stand-off pad or sterile glove filled with water will improve the image by bringing the *superficial* tissues into the probe focal zone (Figs 14.1 and 14.2).

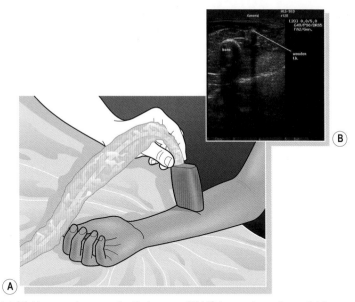

Fig. 14.1 (A) Linear probe on patient's forearm. (B) US image, loss of near field.

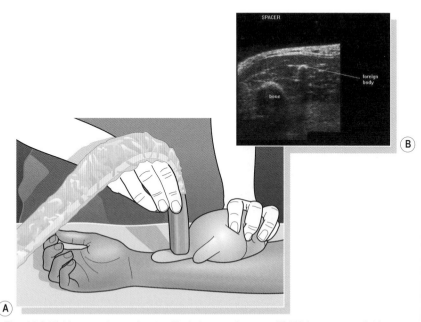

Fig. 14.2 (A) Linear probe and water-filled glove on forearm. (B) US image, near field.

- Deeper FB: 5–7.5 MHz linear array transducer is most useful.
- Focus and depth setting depends on suspected FB depth.

Probe placement and landmarks for FB localization

- Scan along the suspected FB track (Fig. 14.3).
- FBs are usually hyperechoic and often demonstrate posterior shadowing if they are sufficiently dense (Fig. 14.4). They may be surrounded by hypoechoic fluid due to haematoma or abscess.
- If an abnormality or FB is identified, repeat the scan with the probe rotated through 90 degrees and confirm that it conforms to the shape of the suspected FB. Also note if there is more than one FB or if a single piece of wood has broken into several fragments.
- If in doubt about the nature of an identified structure, then scan the same area on the other limb to exclude a normal anatomical structure. Colour Doppler may be of value in distinguishing normal vessels if there is doubt about a structure.
- When an FB is identified, mark it at the skin surface and note any adjacent anatomy, such as vessels, joints or tendons, which may be important during subsequent surgical removal.
- Needle localization may be required to aid removal of an FB.

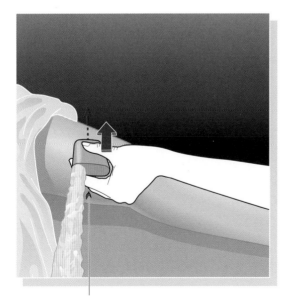

Fig. 14.3 Scanning along FB track.

Entry point of foreign body

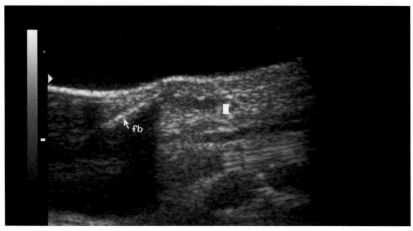

Fig. 14.4 Foreign body (FB) with posterior shadowing, US image.

FB removal

Before proceeding, obtain informed consent, clean the skin with antiseptic and use sterile technique, sterile gel and probe sheath. Once prepared, proceed as follows:

1. Prepare with local anaesthetic.
2. Scan along the suspected FB track. Introduce a fine needle (e.g. 25G) through the skin so that the needle tip or its artefact is visible on the image. Slowly advance the needle until it is in contact with the FB. The needle can then be used to direct surgical intervention.
3. It may be tempting to attempt real-time removal of an FB under US guidance; however, the authors find this impractical for the following reasons:
   - Incising along the wound track introduces air into the soft tissues, obscuring the US image.
   - Scanning and performing the removal simultaneously can be awkward and requires four hands rather than two.

Handy hints

✓ Use a stand-off pad or sterile glove filled with water to improve view of *superficial* tissues.

✓ If in doubt about the nature of an identified structure, scan the same area on the other limb to exclude a normal anatomical structure.

✓ Mark the position of the FB with a pen or needle to aid in subsequent removal.

What US can tell you

- Whether an FB is present.
- Position of an FB.
- Presence of multiple FBs.

- Presence of nearby structures, e.g. tendons, vessels.

What US can't tell you

- Nature of the FB.
- Nature of the surrounding fluid.

 Believe the patient and not the scan. If the patient says that an FB is present it usually is.

Now what?

- US *positive*. Consider FB removal after evaluating symptoms and proximity of important anatomical structures.
- US *negative*. Consider repeating US and evaluating symptoms in approximately 1–2 weeks.

Alternatively, discuss with radiologist regarding further imaging.

- US *positive but undetectable at operation*. Repeat US and guide needle to FB in wound. Dissect along needle towards FB.

 Do not attempt to remove an FB just because it is there. Always consider the patient's wishes and symptoms and the local anatomy.

Summary

➡ US is useful for identifying a soft-tissue FB.
➡ US can identify an FB not seen on plain radiographs.
➡ US can aid FB removal.
➡ US is not an alternative to history and physical examination.

Emergency ultrasound in combat/austere settings

Andrew W Kirkpatrick, John T McManus, Russell McLaughlin

Why use ultrasound in this setting?

- Ultrasound (US) is typically the only diagnostic imaging technology that can be easily transported to many austere and combat settings, and that can be battery-powered.

- Furthermore, US can be used to image widely throughout the body, examining numerous organ systems and structures. Thus, its findings often direct resuscitation and immediate clinical management.

- It can be repeated at will (e.g. if the patient remains unstable despite treatment).

- US easily documents physiology and anatomy digitally which facilitates documentation and telemedicine. Remote interpretation by physically distant experts has been demonstrated in both terrestrial and space settings.

- The scope of this examination theoretically encompasses the entire contents of this book. For practical purposes, therefore, this chapter will emphasize the examinations

most practical to apply to the unstable patient in an austere/combat environment (Fig. 15.1).

Scope of resuscitative US in austere/combat settings

- Airway assessment
- Breathing
  - apnoea
  - haemothorax
  - pneumothorax
  - alveolar-interstitial syndrome
- Circulation
  - death
  - cardiac tamponade
  - hypovolaemia
  - ventricular failure
  - haemoperitoneum
  - vascular access
- Long-bone fractures.

Handy hints and pitfalls

✓ Resuscitative US is very operator dependent. For this reason, it is used to *supplement* the physical assessment, and results must be interpreted with caution.

✓ US results that confirm clinical opinion (e.g. positive focused assessment with sonography in trauma (FAST) in a shocked patient) are most helpful. However, negative or non-diagnostic findings must be interpreted cautiously or even ignored in evaluating the patient.

✓ *Treat the patient, not the picture!*

✓ There is no point in creating delay to scan if the information will not advance clinical care or evacuation.

✓ As fat is an enemy of US, previously fit, healthy subjects typically participating in operational settings are usually well examined by US.

Before you scan

• Ensure the safety and security of the patient/care provider prior to providing medical care (evacuation to shelter/successful firefight/environmental protection from further harm or injury). Becoming a casualty yourself does not benefit your patient.

• Ensure a patent airway.

• Ensure exsanguinating external haemorrhage controlled with direct pressure.

• Triage: with multiple causalities the absence of respiratory activity (bilateral absent lung sliding) and absent cardiac activity (cardiac standstill) precludes resuscitation efforts in the austere/combat setting.

Airway and breathing

See Ch. 5, *Lung and thorax* for detailed description of techniques and findings.

Airway assessment with US

Rationale

• Transport vehicles such as rotary wing aircraft, the International Space Station and active combat zones often preclude the use of the stethoscope due to ambient noise.

• Advanced airway adjuncts such as capnography are typically unavailable.

• Air is a near-complete reflector of US. Therefore, normal lung cannot be seen with US. However, most *rapidly* life-threatening thoracic trauma involves the pleural space rather than the lungs proper.

• Using US, the normal visceral pleura can be seen to 'slide' on the parietal pleura during normal breathing.

• US can be used to facilitate the correct placement of an endotracheal tube (ETT). If the pleura is sliding, the patient is breathing. In an intubated apnoeic or paralysed patient, presence of true pleural sliding on both sides of the chest confirms ETT placement.

Pitfalls

• Sliding gives no indication of the adequacy of ventilation.

- True lung sliding should be distinguished from cardiac oscillations termed the lung pulse.

Breathing assessment with US

Rationale

- Tension pneumothorax (PTX) is a leading cause of preventable death.
- US examination for PTX may safely avoid iatrogenic harm from non-indicated needle thoracocentesis.

Pitfalls

- The lack of lung sliding suggests a PTX but may represent either apnoea or simply pleural fusion/adhesion at that site.

Circulation

See Ch. 4, *FAST and EFAST* and Ch. 6, *Focused echocardiography and volume assessment* for detailed description of techniques and findings.

Rationale

- Haemorrhage is the leading cause of preventable trauma deaths in the world.
- Major haemoperitoneum is relatively frequent with intra-abdominal trauma, while the absence of a haemoperitoneum in conjunction with a major pelvic fracture suggests retroperitoneal bleeding.

- Gross ventricular function can often be categorically determined with US.
- Cardiac standstill can be easily distinguished from relatively normal or vigorous pumping and from a failing ventricle with modest experience.
- In the austere setting, US is helpful for triage decisions such as determining who to evacuate first, by what method, or who is beyond salvage, depending on the circumstances.

Pitfalls

- If the FAST exam is indeterminate, it is usually unhelpful to repeat the exam and another approach should be used.

Musculoskeletal

See Ch. 13, *Musculoskeletal and soft tissues* for detailed description of techniques and findings.

Rationale

- Normally bony injuries are not life-threatening. In an operational setting, however, a bony injury may threaten the lives of the individual and the team, as well as the mission itself.
- Highly motivated individuals will often deny/be unaware of serious performance-limiting injuries.
- Confirmation of a fracture can justify complex extractions or mission delay/termination.

Technique

- Typically a high-frequency linear transducer is used to image the bony cortex in both the transverse and longitudinal planes.
- If there is any doubt as to the presence of a cortical defect, the normal contralateral extremity should be used as the comparison.

Pitfalls

- While long bone shafts are typically easily imaged, the diaphyses, and small bones of the extremities, and joints require significant operator experience.

Telemedicine using US in austere settings

- US is the only diagnostic imaging modality on board the International Space Station, and thus has been incorporated into nearly all treatment algorithms on board.
- As experienced ultrasonographers are typically unavailable in space, NASA has led the development of telemedical techniques using ground-based experts to guide the less experienced onboard examiners.
- Remote telementoring is satisfactory in remote terrestrial settings.

Future directions

- US is increasingly frequently carried in transport and resuscitative vehicles and will likely be an indispensable personal tool in the next decade.
- US will become increasingly cheap yet more powerful and user-friendly. Hundreds of US units could be purchased for the developed world for the same cost as advanced CT and MRI equipment.
- Solar-powered US will be ideal for the developing world.
- Remote telemedicine support and robotic examinations are becoming available.
- Decision-support and auto-interpretation will likely be increasingly available.
- Most importantly, all medical students will learn US as a basic skill automatically integrated into the physical examination.

16 Conclusion

Russell McLaughlin, Justin Bowra

We hope that you have found this book enjoyable and instructive. It cannot be stressed enough that:

- This book does not represent an exhaustive text of ultrasound (US). However, the reader should bear in mind that the emergency sonologist does not require an exhaustive knowledge of all aspects of US.

- While this book represents one approach to the role of critical care US, there will be other perfectly valid practices.

As noted in Chapter 1, the critical care sonologist simply requires the knowledge and skills required to perform emergency procedural US and to answer the basic questions raised in each chapter. The aim of this chapter is to summarize key areas to address when considering critical care US on an individual and departmental basis.

Audit/quality control/training

The authors recommend that the practice of critical care US is learned and practised in a formal and structured manner including the following.

Audit and quality control

All US images should be reviewed for diagnostic quality and correct patient disposal on a regular basis. In the first edition of this textbook we recommended that this should occur as a joint exercise between the lead critical care clinician and a radiology colleague, but this advice is less practical given that critical care US has expanded to 'non-radiologist' areas such as nerve block and echocardiography. The principle remains the same: the lead clinician should retain close contacts with a broad cross-section of experts in each field of critical care US practised by the department.

As expertise in critical care US develops, the specialties of emergency medicine and intensive care medicine will become more autonomous in terms of quality assurance and governance.

Training

All clinicians engaged in training should be enrolled in a structured programme including supervised US practice, formal teaching and periodic summative assessments of their skills in image acquisition and interpretation. This process is by no means standardized; however, it is the responsibility of the practitioner to agree on and achieve an acceptable standard of practice in keeping with local policy where national policy does not exist.

Managerial

It is the responsibility of the lead clinician/departmental manger to consider the broader issues relating to critical care US. These are as follows:

- Political. The most important issue here is the relationship with the other departments which perform US on site (e.g. radiology, vascular surgery, cardiology). It is also vital that other stakeholders are aware of the limitations and benefits of the technology. For example, it is vital that surgical colleagues are prepared to act on information given (e.g. abdominal aortic aneurysm (AAA), abdominal fluid, and hip effusion).
- Capital and revenue costs including business case development for US machine.

Research and future directions

Like all areas of clinical practice, it is important for clinicians to keep abreast of research and future developments in their own field and to implement evidence-based practice. Some clinicians may wish to engage in research and use point-of-care US as a useful tool.

The concept of 'old technology–new application' has driven much of the recent evolution of critical care US, as have the advances in portable machine technology. Furthermore, the sheer number of clinicians who are embracing US in their practice will continue to test the limits of this tool. For these reasons, critical care US will continue to evolve rapidly. For example, the use of lung US to diagnose pulmonary oedema was dismissed as speculative until fairly recently, and contrast-enhanced US is generating international interest in the investigation of abdominal trauma.

Research regarding emergency department (ED) US can be stratified into a number of levels:

- Technological/cutting edge: for example, improved computer technology, US contrast, smaller US machines, three-dimensional (3-D) and four-dimensional (4-D) US. It is likely that this research will come from the US manufacturers and research radiologists/scientists. There will probably be a significant lag phase of years before any useful ED application evolves.
- Clinical trials: for example, focused assessment with sonography in trauma (FAST), AAA. There is good research from a number of centres worldwide on the benefits of these

applications in the ED. However, users must first critically appraise the evidence in terms of their own local setting.

- Local validation studies: for example, introducing a new application such as first trimester scanning, biliary scanning. There is a role for introducing new applications based on evidence from other centres.

 A fool with a stethoscope will still be a fool with US.

Summary

- All of the above issues must be considered before embarking on critical care US practice.
- The practitioner must be aware of the clinical and political issues and place the clinical condition of the patient above all.
- Critical care US will never replace sound clinical judgement.

1 Appendix

Useful paperwork: logbook sheet

Sample ED ultrasound log

Adapted with permission from Emergency Department, Royal North Shore Hospital, Sydney, Australia

Patient's details *(or apply sticker)*

ED ultrasonographer (name & signature)..

....

Date & time ....

Indication ....

Views: *(tick as appropriate)*	**YES**	**NO**	**Poorly visualized**
Free fluid in abdomen	❑	❑	❑
Free fluid in thorax	❑	❑	❑
Pneumothorax	❑	❑	❑
Pericardial fluid	❑	❑	❑
Cardiac abnormal (details) . . . . ❑		❑	❑
Abdominal aortic aneurysm	❑	❑	❑
GB/CBD abnormal: details . . . . ❑		❑	❑
Renal tract abnormal: details . . . . ❑		❑	❑
Deep venous thrombosis above knee	❑	❑	❑
Hip effusion	❑	❑	❑
Other (details) . . . . ❑		❑	❑

Images saved?   ❑ **YES**   ❑ **NO**

Hard copy?   ❑ **YES**   ❑ **NO**   *(please staple to this sheet)*

Ultrasound diagnosis & time made: . . . .

Final clinical diagnosis & time made: . . . .

Basis of final diagnosis (e.g. CT): . . . .

Radiologist/Senior EM review: name . . . . date. . . . .

Adequate images?   ❑ **YES**   ❑ **NO**

If Yes, correct interpretation?   ❑ **YES**   ❑ **NO**

Other diagnostic procedures:

	Confirm diagnosis	**Refute diagnosis**	**Comment**
CT	❑	❑	
Operation	❑	❑	
Other (e.g. angiogram)	❑	❑	

2 Appendix

Useful organizations

Up-to-date credentialing and specialty-specific information and guidelines are available from the following organizations. This is by no means an exclusive or exhaustive list of contacts in emergency ultrasound.

United States of America

- American College of Emergency Physicians (ACEP)
  - www.acep.org
- American College of Radiology (ACR)
  - www.acr.org
- American Institute of Ultrasound in Medicine (AIUM)
  - www.aium.org

Australasia

- Australasian College for Emergency Medicine
  - www.acem.org.au
- Australasian Society for Ultrasound in Medicine (ASUM)
  - www.asum.com.au

United Kingdom

- The College of Emergency Medicine
  - www.collemergencymed.ac.uk
- British Medical Ultrasound Society
  - www.bmus.org
- Royal College of Radiologists
  - www.rcr.ac.uk

3 Appendix

Further reading

Beebe HG, Kritpracha B 2003 Imaging of abdominal aortic aneurysm: current status. Annals of Vascular Surgery 17:111–118.

Brenchley J, Sloan JP, Thompson PK 2000 Echoes of things to come: ultrasound in UK Emergency Medical Practice. Journal of Accident and Emergency Medicine 17:170–175.

Broos PLO, Gutermann H 2002 Actual diagnostic strategies in blunt abdominal trauma. European Journal of Trauma 2:64–74.

Burnett HC, Nicholson DA 1999 Current and future role of ultrasound in the Emergency Department. Journal of Accident and Emergency Medicine 16:250–254.

Dart RG, Kaplan B, Cox C 1997 Transvaginal ultrasound in patients with low beta-human chorionic gonadotrophin values: how often is the study diagnostic? Annals of Emergency Medicine 30(2):135–140.

Durston W, Carl ML, Guerra W 1999 Patient satisfaction and diagnostic accuracy with ultrasound by emergency physicians. American Journal of Emergency Medicine 17(7): 642–646.

Feigenbaum H 1994 Echocardiography, 5th edn. Lea & Febiger, Baltimore, ISBN 0 8121 1692 5.

Gent R 1997 Applied physics and technology of diagnostic ultrasound. Miner Publishing, Prospect, South Australia, ISBN 0646276018.

Hagen-Ansert SL 1989 Textbook of diagnostic ultrasonography, 3rd edn. Mosby, London, ISBN 0 8016 2446 0.

Heller M, Jehle D 1997 Ultrasound in emergency: out of the acoustic shadow. Annals of Emergency Medicine 29:380–382.

Holmes JF, Harris D, Baltiselle FD 2003 Performance of abdominal ultrasonography in blunt trauma patients with out of hospital or emergency department hypotension. Annals of Emergency Medicine 43(3):354–361.

Jolly BT, Massarin E, Pigman EC 1997 Colour Doppler ultrasonography by emergency physicians for the diagnosis of acute deep venous thrombosis. Academic Emergency Medicine 4:129–132.

Kaddoura S 2002 Echo made easy. Churchill Livingstone, Edinburgh, ISBN 0 443 06188 2.

Kuhn M, Bonnin RL, Davey MJ et al 2000 Emergency department ultrasound scanning for abdominal aortic aneurysm: accessible, accurate, and advantageous. Annals of Emergency Medicine 36(3):219–223.

Lanoix R, Baker WE, Mele JM, Dharmarajan L 1998 Evaluation of an instructional model for emergency ultrasonography. Academic Emergency Medicine 5(1):58–63.

Lichtenstein DA 2002 General ultrasound in the critically ill. Springer, ISBN 3-540-20822-4.

Ma OJ, Mateer J R 2003 Emergency ultrasound. McGraw-Hill, New York, ISBN 0 071 37417 5.

Ma OJ, Mateer JR, Ogata M et al 1995 Prospective analysis of a rapid trauma ultrasound examination performed by emergency physicians. Journal of Trauma 38(6):879–885.

Mandavia DP, Aragona J, Chan L 2000 Ultrasound training for emergency physicians—a prospective study. Academic Emergency Medicine 7(9):1008–1014.

Mateer J, Valley V, Aiman E et al 1996 Outcome analysis of a protocol including bedside endovaginal sonography in patients at risk for ectopic pregnancy. Annals of Emergency Medicine 27:283–289.

McMinn RMH 1994 Last's anatomy, 9th edn. Churchill Livingstone, Edinburgh, ISBN 0 443 04662 X.

Nilsson A 2002 Knowledge of artefacts helps prevent errors. Diagnostic Imaging Europe December 25–29.

Royal College of Radiologists, Faculty of Clinical Radiologists 2005 Ultrasound training recommendations for medical and surgical specialties. London.

Rumack CM, Wilson SR, Charboneau JW 2004 Diagnostic ultrasound, 3rd edn. Mosby, ISBN 0 323 02023 2.

Schlager D 1997 Ultrasound detection of foreign bodies and procedure guidance. Emergency Medicine Clinics of North America 15:895–912.

Shih CHY 1997 Effect of emergency physician-performed pelvic sonography on length of stay in the Emergency Department. Annals of Emergency Medicine 29:348–352.

Sirlin CB, Brown MA, Deutsch R et al 2003 Screening ultrasound for blunt abdominal trauma: objective predictor of false negative findings and missed injury. Radiology 229:766–774.

Taylor Kenneth JW 1985 Atlas of obstetric, gynecologic and perinatal ultrasonography, 2nd edn. Churchill Livingstone, Edinburgh, ISBN 0 443 08443 2.

Index

Page numbers followed by "f" indicate figures, "t" indicate tables, and "b" indicate boxes.

A

A lines, 46
Abdominal aorta, 17–25
  anatomy, 17, 18f
  diameter, 17, 18f, 22–23, 23f–24f
  differentiation from inferior vena cava, 19, 21t, 23, 25f
  ecstatic, 23, 24f
  essential views, 22, 22f
Abdominal aortic aneurysm (AAA), 1, 17
  clinical picture, 17–19
  leaking, 23
  rupture, 17, 23
  scanning technique/views, 19–22
    essential views, 22, 22f
    patient position, 19
    probe placement and landmarks, 19–21, 20f–21f
    probe/scanner settings, 19
    stable patient, 25
    unstable patient, 25, 74
Abscess, 124f, 170–174, 174f
Acetabulum, 167
Acoustic enhancement, 12, 13f
Acoustic impedance, 7
Acoustic shadowing, 12, 13f–14f
Acoustic windows, 12
Acromioclavicular arch, 175
Acute renal failure (ARF), 75, 84
Adnexal mass, 106
Age-related multicystic kidney disease, 82
Airway and breathing, resuscitative ultrasound, 190–191
Alcoholic cardiomyopathy, 66–67
Alveolar consolidation, 53
Alveolar-interstitial syndrome, 51
Anaemia, 68

Anisotropy, 135, 137f
Aortic dissection, 23, 26f
Apical view
  focused echocardiography, 64, 65f
Artefacts, 11–15
  see also specific types
Arteries
  distinguishing from nerves, 134–135
  distinguishing from veins, 121
Arthrocentesis, 168–169
Ascites, 124f
Audit, 195–196
Austere settings *see* Combat/austere settings, ultrasound in
Axillary artery, 145
Axillary block, 134, 145, 145f–147f, 150

B

B lines, 46–47, 47f, 51, 54
β-human chorionic gonadotropin (βHCG), 100–101
Biliary colic, 96
Binary thinking, 2, 2t
Bladder, 35–36, 78
  echogenicity, 8f
  position, 76–78
  reverberation artefact, 15f
  scanning technique, 83
Bladder outlet obstruction, 75
Blood echogenicity, 41
B-mode, 5
Bone
  echogenicity, 7, 7f–8f
  injuries, 192
  ultrasound appearance, 172
Bowel gas, 22, 123
Brachial plexus, 134, 134f, 142–145
Breathing, resuscitative ultrasound, 190–191
Breathlessness, 44, 55

Index